T0017555

An Illustrated Instruction Manual for
FIRST-TIME FATHERS

HOW TO
DAD

WRITTEN AND ILLUSTRATED BY
T.M. DETWILER

Dedicated to my dad,

Thomas F. Detwiler Jr., for showing me how to hold a pencil
and draw the world around me.

TABLE OF CONTENTS

Because you'll
need a break from
all this baby talk

DAD TIPS

Here's a tip: Don't be
afraid to try something
new. Experience will give
you the confidence to
fake like you're an expert
with your kids.

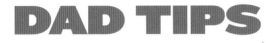

An Introduction

FROM THE DAD WHO WROTE THIS BOOK

→ Because it's always important to know what kind of well the water is coming from.

BEFORE THIS BOOK WAS even a germ of an idea, I found out I was going to be a father. I was thrilled. I felt ready (relatively) and couldn't wait to go to every doctor's appointment and prepare for the baby's arrival. I was engaged in every moment, immersed myself in as much intel as I could find and when labor finally began, I knew I was ready. I was wrong. After nine months of pregnancy and a year with a baby, it became obvious to me the resources available to new parents, while informative, can be tough to digest (you also don't have a ton of time to read when you're in the middle of dealing with a diaper blowout). Like a lot of people, I'm a visual learner. I'm also a visual communicator (if I could have drawn this intro, I would have). To me, an illustrated guide to fatherhood felt like a home run. So I set out to create the book I wished I'd had when I was an eager-to-learn but not eager-to-read father.

I suspect there are plenty of dads out there who can relate to the struggle. We want to have all the info we can. We're interested in being a dad: Burping the baby and building the crib and changing the diapers (as much as anyone can be, anyway). We want to know what to expect, but we also want to know how we can be helpful. Useful. Or at least not in the way. Dads quickly find out they are the fourth most important person in the room (at best) when it comes to pregnancy. It's a mom-only journey physically, which is why it is important to find moments when you can be exemplary. Your pursuit of papa perfection will extend

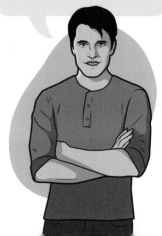

"I hope you enjoy what's written here and find it useful as you begin your journey into fatherhood. There is no greater responsibility or reward."

—T.M. DETWILER

beyond your child's time in utero, which is theoretically why you're consulting this book.

But here's the thing: This book is not perfect. Like a lot of guidebooks, you may not even feel you need it. You may think, like I did, you've got this thing nailed and everything will go as you've planned. But then the baby arrives and the plans you've made shift dramatically and you find yourself Googling "how to swaddle" at 3 a.m. because you can't figure out how to secure your baby's incessantly wriggling form. Plans change.

Neither of my kids' deliveries were textbook. In fact, both spent some time in the NICU. I got to witness an emergency C-section when our daughter was born six weeks early (the hospital staff went from semi-casual and friendly to the "not-effin-around" crew in a blink). Like I said, plans change.

To create the guidebook I always wanted, I did a great deal of research beyond my own experience and leaned on experts to provide the most medically sound advice available. Regardless of that work, you may find this book doesn't have every answer to every question on your mind.

Always consult your physician and embrace your gut instincts even as you embrace the dad bod.

The moment you take your baby home from the hospital, all the stories you've heard about fatherhood start happening to you. The first few weeks are a bit of a blur, and they go by quickly. Take time to reflect on these moments and understand that this is the smallest your child will ever be. You'll eventually find a rhythm, and just when you're in a great groove, the kid changes the game. You'll make more plans. Those plans will change. This book will be here when they do.

Writing this book felt a bit like having our first baby. There were a number of setbacks, some tears and a lot of long nights. But I wouldn't trade a moment. I feel so lucky to be a father. Each day, my kids grow bigger and stronger, speak new words, ask new questions, run a little faster. I can already feel them starting to become individuals with their own thoughts and opinions. It's a magical feeling, and I hope it never ends. My plans may change. The joy of fatherhood will not.

Welcome to the club.

—Todd

Before We Begin...

Before any arduous journey, it's
wise to get the lay of the land.
In this case, the land is your baby.
Here's a basic map.

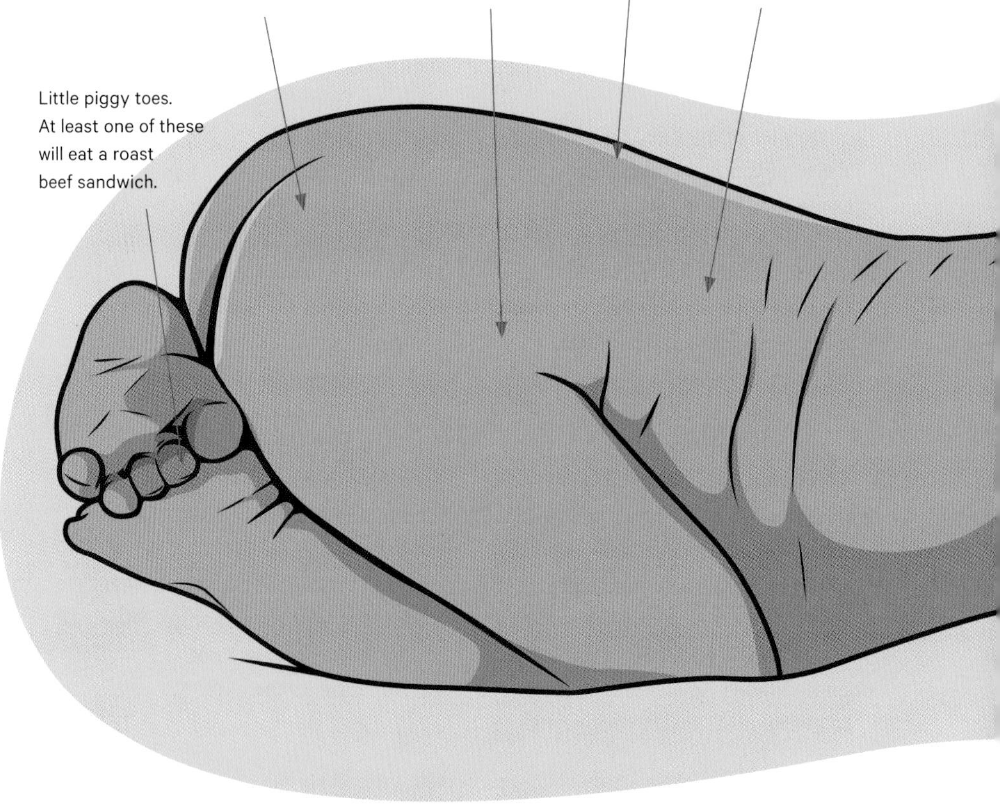

A baby's skin is
sensitive, because, ya
know, it's brand new.
Treat it like Cameron's
dad treated that Ferrari.

A baby's stomach
grows from the
size of a marble to
the size of a ping-
pong ball in the
first 10 days.

Babies smell good,
except maybe around
these parts. But they
clean up quick.

For the first few
weeks, baby might
have froggy legs from
being cooped up in the
womb for months.

Little piggy toes.
At least one of these
will eat a roast
beef sandwich.

Baby's eyes might not open right away. Once they do, they may go in opposite directions, like a chameleon. This is normal.

Baby's head has soft spots for several weeks after birth. They're part of the skull where formation is not complete so the skull can be molded during birth. Don't press them.

Some babies are born with a lot of hair, some babies have none. Either way, they get a hat upon arrival.

Baby's neck (and head for that matter) will need extra support until they're strong enough to hold their melon up by themselves.

Baby's are cute and people like to hold them. You have a right to be discerning.

THE END GOAL
This is what you're working toward: a baby! They're cute, they're fun, they're a lot of work. You'll be ready. You've got this book.

Chapter 1

HOW WE GOT HERE

These first 12 weeks of pregnancy will see your baby grow and change from a twinkle in your eye to about the size of a plum. Take this time to get a jump on your new gig as Dad by reflecting on what your upcoming task will look like.

A Brief History of Dad

For the first few hundred thousand years of human (and pre-human) history, our hunter-gatherer ancestors divided tasks evenly amongst members of the large clannish groups in which they moved. According to anthropologists like Sebastian Kraemer, who wrote the 1991 paper "The Origins of Fatherhood: An Ancient Family Process," in these groups men communally hunted game while women communally performed the dual tasks of gathering plant-based foods and caring for the group's youngest members. It wasn't until the Neolithic Revolution—when these hunter-gatherer groups first began harvesting crops and domesticating livestock, allowing them to remain in one place rather than roam the land in search of their next meal—that the role of dad as we know it came into being. Over the next few millennia, each new change in civilization has ushered in an evolution in the very idea of "dad," and that's not just in the facial hair department.

1776
Revolutionary-era dad stuck to old-world ideals, deriving his dad playbook from the Bible and the lessons his own father had imparted. Many of these lessons involved negative reinforcement.

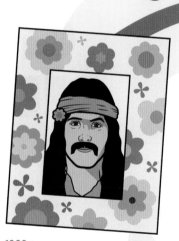

1960s
As more and more moms flock to offices and job sites in a wave of cultural revolution, the scale of responsibility in child rearing begins, at long last, to balance. Cue the "Mr. Mom" jokes.

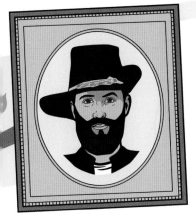

1865
Industrialization sweeps across America following the division wrought by the Civil War. For a time, this means many fathers and sons labor together side by side in their trades for long hours with no PTO.

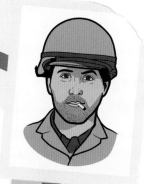

1941–1945
As the U.S. enters World War II, fathers and sons from all over the country risk everything in the hopes of ending fascism forever and making the world safe for dad jokes—and democracy.

1950s
Suburban dads learn that interstate highways give them an excuse for endless family road trips. The dawn of television helps repopularize the notion that Father Knows Best.

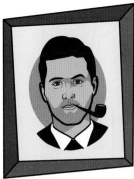

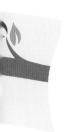

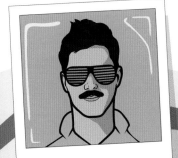

MODERN DAD
COVID-19 redefines dad's role yet again, ushering in the era of "Take Your Daughter To Work Everyday."

1977
The Atari 2600 gaming console ushers in an era for dads in which we don't have to leave the couch to prove to our kids that we are superior at all sports and games.

Pregnancy Tests

These nifty tubes of plastic measure a hormone in the body called human chorionic gonadotropin (hCG). This is produced during pregnancy and appears in the blood and urine of pregnant women as early as 10 days after conception. Most over-the-counter tests are 99 percent reliable, so you should take the results seriously (even if you or your partner insist on throwing more than one into your shopping cart). For simplicity's sake, use the ones that clearly state "PREGNANT" or "NOT PREGNANT."

Stand back and let Mom do her thing according to the instructions and wait for the recommended amount of time. Remember to breathe.

................wait for it................

................wait for it................

CONGRATS! YOUR LIFE IS FOREVER CHANGED!

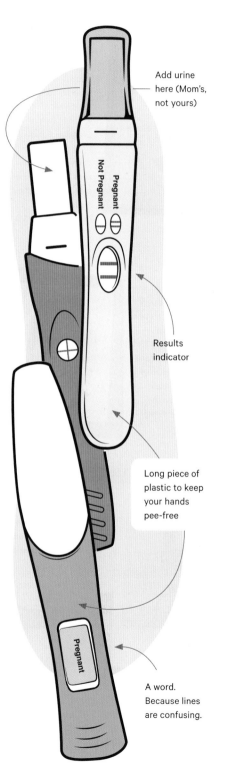

Add urine here (Mom's, not yours)

Results indicator

Long piece of plastic to keep your hands pee-free

A word. Because lines are confusing.

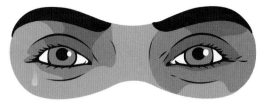

Your Reaction!

There's no telling exactly how you'll respond to some of the most important news of your life, but it's important to remember your reaction will affect others and possibly be burned into their memories for all time.

If you've already reacted to the pregnancy test, see if you can find your face on the page. How'd you do?

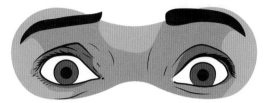

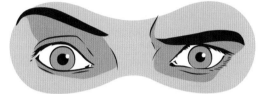

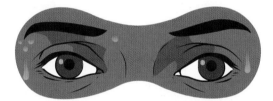

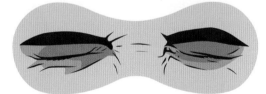

MAKE IT COUNT

Whether the pregnancy is expected or a surprise, this is a moment that will speak to your character.

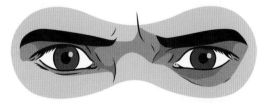

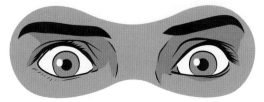

What to Eat

You might not have officially stepped into your role as Dad just yet, but one thing's for sure: You are what you eat. That's especially true for Mom while she's pregnant and nursing. Keep each other in good health throughout the pregnancy by sticking to meals and snacks that are high in protein, vegetables, healthy fats and fiber-rich carbohydrates. A healthy diet is important throughout your life, and a pregnancy is a great reason to get yourself back on track as you both prepare to raise a healthy child.

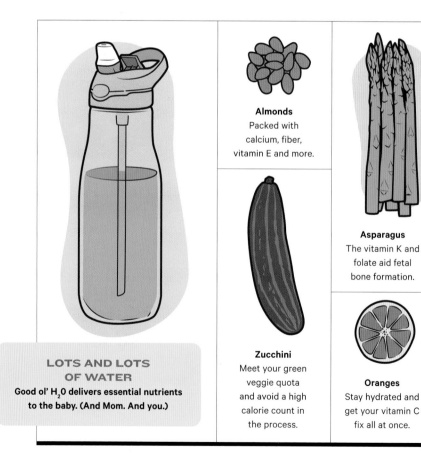

LOTS AND LOTS OF WATER
Good ol' H₂O delivers essential nutrients to the baby. (And Mom. And you.)

Almonds
Packed with calcium, fiber, vitamin E and more.

Zucchini
Meet your green veggie quota and avoid a high calorie count in the process.

Asparagus
The vitamin K and folate aid fetal bone formation.

Oranges
Stay hydrated and get your vitamin C fix all at once.

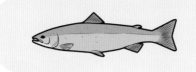

SALMON

The safest seafood choice for pregnant women, this fish is rich in DHA, which is important for neurodevelopment.

Bell Peppers
Helps reduce the risk of high blood pressure.

Blueberries
A great snack and source for antioxidants.

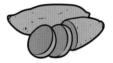

Bananas
Loaded with potassium.

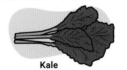

Sweet potatoes
Low in fat, rich in antioxidants, fiber and potassium.

Apples
Full of vitamins A and C and fiber.

Broccoli
Full of fiber, which prevents constipation (which... she'll want to do).

Kale
A pregnancy superfood packed with vitamins, iron and fiber.

Black beans
Rich in zinc, which keeps the immune system strong.

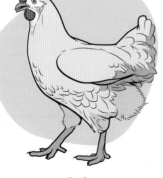

Poultry
Excellent source of lean protein.

Avocados
Regulates blood sugar and can protect against pregnancy complications.

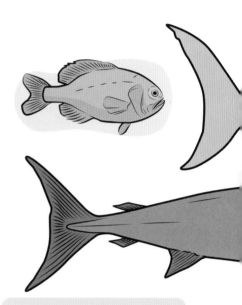

What *Not* to Eat

Mom will need to be mindful of not only the best foods to eat but also the ones she should avoid entirely. While Dad can still technically eat whatever the hell he wants, a little solidarity goes a long way. Learn which foods are on the no-go list so you can support your partner and give her one less thing to worry about (and she'll have plenty).

HIGH-MERCURY FISH
This includes swordfish, tuna, bass and orange roughy. The mercury in these fish can negatively affect the baby's development.

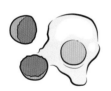

Raw eggs
Sorry, no *Rocky* montages. Cook any eggs to raise "good" cholesterol levels.

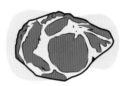

Undercooked meat
Still mooing (or oinking) meats can harbor bacteria that might make you sick and cause complications.

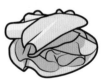

Processed meat
These may contain listeria, a serious threat that could cause a miscarriage.

ALCOHOL

No alcohol of any kind is a good rule of thumb. Some Dads-to-be go sober with Mom for 9 months...not for everybody.

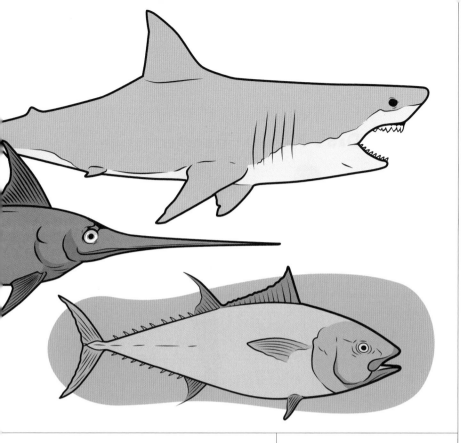

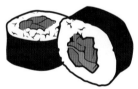

Sushi (raw)
See undercooked meat. However, an avocado or California roll is perfectly fine!

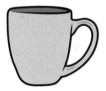

Caffeine
A cup a day might be OK, provided "one cup" doesn't mean Venti double red-eye with extra cream.

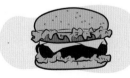

Junk food
Pregnancy is definitely the wrong time to raise your cholesterol and blood pressure. Our fatty faves do both.

Sprouts
While seemingly healthy, raw sprouts of any sort can host harmful bacteria. Skip them.

Mom's and Dad's Physical Transformation

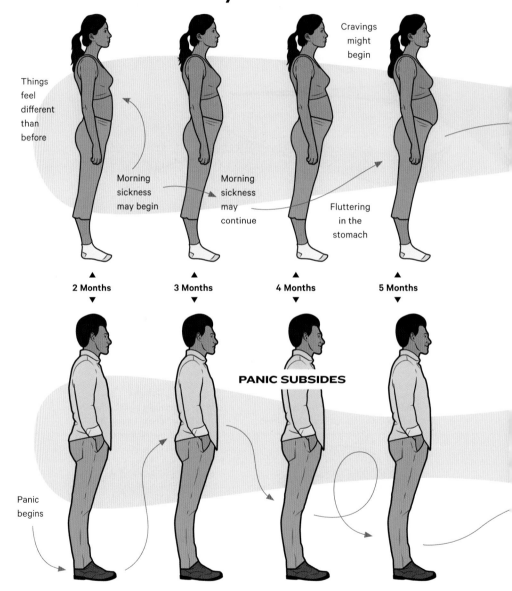

Things feel different than before

Cravings might begin

Morning sickness may begin

Morning sickness may continue

Fluttering in the stomach

2 Months **3 Months** **4 Months** **5 Months**

PANIC SUBSIDES

Panic begins

There's a moment right about here where Dad says "I'm going to get back into shape before baby arrives." AND YOU SHOULD!

Should have learned how to give an incredible foot massage (pg. 38)

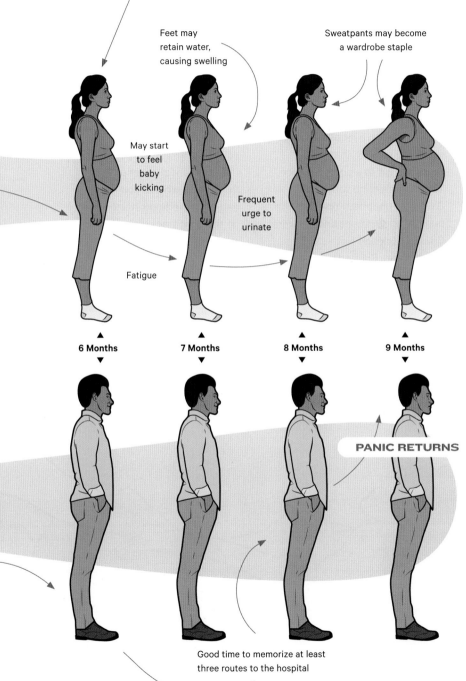

NOTICEABLY PREGNANT!

Feet may retain water, causing swelling

Sweatpants may become a wardrobe staple

May start to feel baby kicking

Frequent urge to urinate

Fatigue

▲ 6 Months ▼

▲ 7 Months ▼

▲ 8 Months ▼

▲ 9 Months ▼

PANIC RETURNS

Good time to memorize at least three routes to the hospital

First Doctor's Visit

We're going to be up-front about this: You should prepare to get clobbered with a lot of information when you roll into that first prenatal visit to a doctor's office. Your first meeting with an OB-GYN is an important one, and the number of questions and answers flowing back and forth can be intimidating. But don't worry—you've got this.

First, you'll want to take care of logistics: Are you and your partner using her regular OB-GYN or finding a new doctor? How much is your copay? You know, all the super fun questions that predate any doctor's visit. Next, get out a pen and paper (or your notepad app) and write down the following: Your family medical history, with special emphasis on any prenatal or neonatal conditions that might be in your family tree, and a list of any questions that pop into your head as you prepare for this visit (cheat sheet at right). Remember, when it comes to getting fatherhood started out on the right track, there are no stupid questions.

While your partner lays on her back with a wand between her thighs, your job is to sit up straight, try to avoid distraction and become a sponge. Absorb all the information you can. Take notes to help you remember important milestones, side effects, remedies, warning signs and anything else that seems important as your partner and her doctor hash out the details. You're the third wheel here, but you're the third wheel on your kid's first tricycle, so your role is important too! Don't be afraid to ask questions if you have them, just remember you're likely to feel like the fourth most important person in the room. But Ringo Starr was a hell of a drummer. Know your role and crush it.

FIRST VISIT
BASIC QUESTIONS

1. Should we research prenatal classes or will you recommend some to us later?

2. When will the next appointment be?

3. Can we travel? How much? Until when?

4. Are there any supplements or prenatal vitamins we should take?

5. Anything we should be on the lookout for based on our medical histories?

6. Is this really happening?

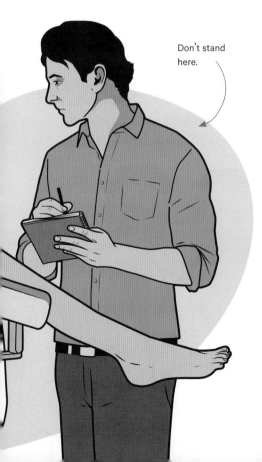

Don't stand here.

Preparing for Bad News

Research suggests 10 to 30 percent of pregnancies end in miscarriage, and of that number, 80 percent happen during the first trimester. If there is no detectable heartbeat by the time Mom has her first vaginal ultrasound around 8 weeks, it's likely (though not certain) that you've suffered a non-viable pregnancy/miscarriage. Frankly, Dad, understanding you could get bad news here is about all you can do to prepare for it. Hang in there.

Interviewing Doctors

Finding the right OB-GYN is a lot like dating but with far fewer apps and far more eligible doctors. You should have a few candidates, a basic understanding of what you're looking for and an open mind in terms of expertise. Definitely don't go with someone simply because a friend recommended them—get to know your doctor first. Here are a few questions to ask along the way.

1. Can we meet your partners?

If your OB-GYN has partners, it's a good idea to get acquainted with them before Mom's water breaks, especially if someone can't make it the day she goes into labor.

2. Will we have a private room?

Many new moms, particularly in larger cities, share rooms with other mothers after their delivery. If this does not sound enjoyable to you or Mom, that's the sort of thing you'll want to know as far ahead of time as possible.

3. Do you accept my insurance?

Let's face it: Delivering a baby is expensive. Every little bit helps.

4. How long are appointments?

Each appointment will have important updates, from hearing the baby's heartbeat to being quietly asked if you "want to know" details that might help you narrow down your list of potential names. You never want to feel like you're in a time crunch.

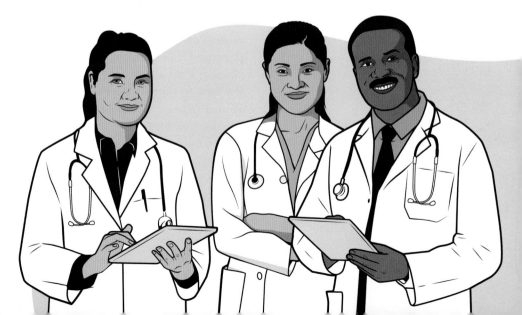

5. Do you have experience with higher risk deliveries?

Preeclampsia, a serious blood pressure condition, is just one of many pregnancy complications women may experience. You want to feel at ease with your doctor's expertise when it comes to dealing with complex situations.

6. Are you open to facilitating our birth plan?

Some women may want the epidural right away, while others may want to deliver naturally. Some want a doula, and others doulanot. Ensuring your doctor is comfortable with what you and your partner want—especially if it's a little "non-traditional"—is a key part of the search for the right doc. Get a feel for the doctor's communication style and overall bedside manner.

GOOD ADVICE FROM A MOM:

Find out their suggested/available interventions in an array of "what if" scenarios: "What if I am 10 days past EDD (estimated due date)?" "What if I have gestational diabetes?"
—BRITTANY B.

What happens if they are on vacation when I deliver or out of town? If so, who would be delivering in their place?
—ALISHA L.

How long will it take for the incision to heal, and is it true I can't pick up my baby while I'm healing?
—TRACEY K.

When looking at hospitals, take tours and ask about what happens when you arrive at the hospital, if they offer pre-payment, how many visitors are allowed, etc.
—KATIE F.

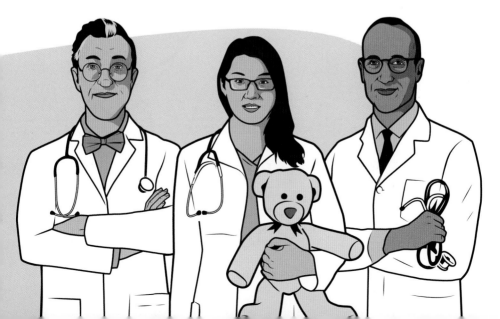

Visualizing Baby's Growth

It isn't called "the miracle of life" for nothing. Here's what your baby looks like during different stages of in-womb development. From the moment of conception, they grow up quick, so don't blink.

On the Microscopic Level:

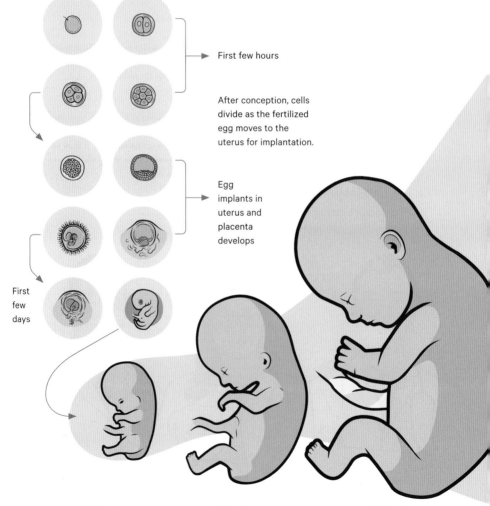

First few hours

After conception, cells divide as the fertilized egg moves to the uterus for implantation.

Egg implants in uterus and placenta develops

First few days

12 Weeks   19 Weeks   24 Weeks

DID YOU KNOW?
The first sense your baby develops is touch. Touch receptors appear as early as 8 weeks!

The lungs are the last organ to develop. As a result, if the baby is pre-term, the lungs will be closely monitored at birth.

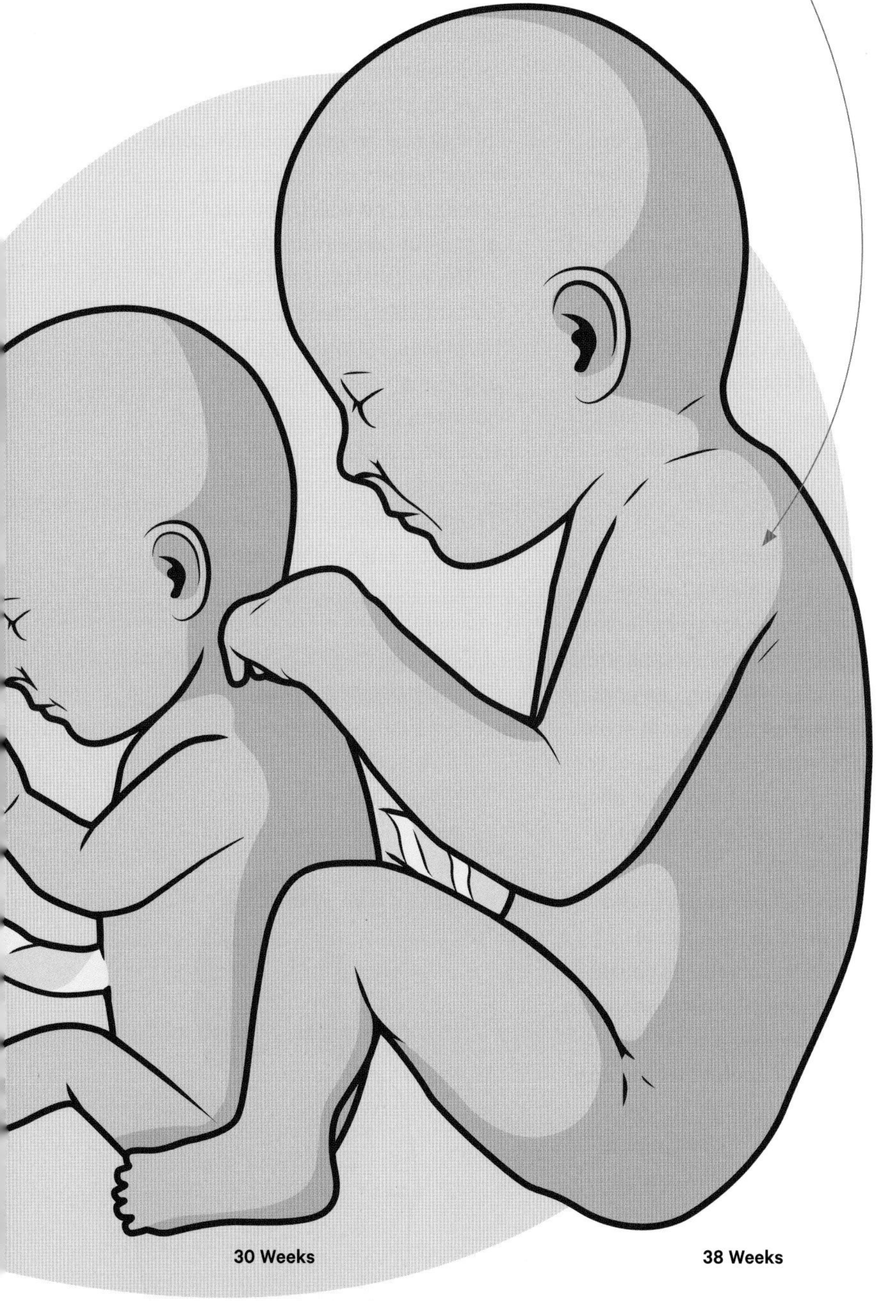

30 Weeks

38 Weeks

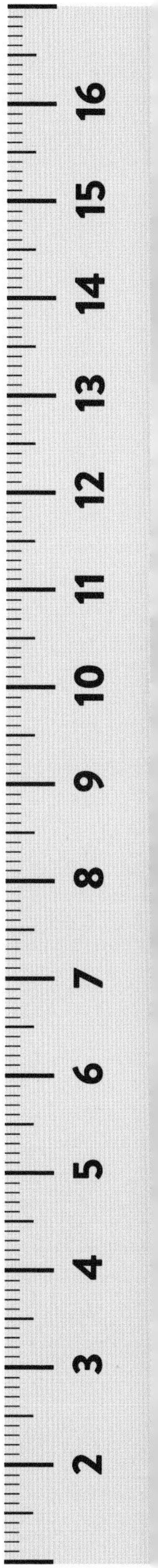

16
15
14
13
12
11
10
9
8
7
6
5
4
3
2

First Trimester Ailments and Solutions

It should go without saying, but having a baby isn't exactly like pulling a rabbit out of a hat (even if the gift of life is pretty magical). If you think your baby's rapid stages of growth are amazing, consider how your partner's body has to shift into human incubator mode in just a few short weeks to accommodate her internal organs shifting over the course of nine months.

The first trimester of pregnancy—a mere 13 weeks—lays the groundwork for an incredible transformation. Mom's appearance and overall well-being can endure any number of changes. In some cases, she will deal with all of them. You get to watch! And hear about it. Your job is to listen and help however you can.

At conception, the fertilized egg implants in the uterine lining (which sometimes causes spotting), its cells rapidly dividing, and by three weeks after the moment your sperm met her egg, voilà: an embryo has formed! This little mass of cells means business: It isn't just going to grow into your baby, it will also develop a placenta—to provide the fetus with nutrients, filter waste from its blood and protect it from infections—and an umbilical cord, which tethers the fetus to the placenta (and which you might just get to cut on delivery day).

The cells that create the placenta also create a surge of hormones: estrogen, progesterone and human chorionic gonadotropin hormone (hCG), which triggered that "PREGNANT" result on the pregnancy test (see pg. 18). These hormones pave the way for your little one's safe development

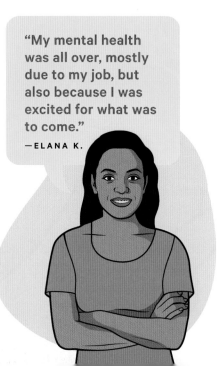

"My mental health was all over, mostly due to my job, but also because I was excited for what was to come."

—ELANA K.

but also wreak havoc on Mom's body and mood.

Collectively, these hormones send signals throughout your partner's body: to stop ovulating, increase blood flow, increase the thickness of the uterine lining, provide nutrients to the growing embryo, prep the mammary glands for making breast milk and much more. Unfortunately, the sudden rise of these hormones can also cause Mom to experience a bevy of unpleasant side effects.

Her breasts, for example, might feel swollen, sensitive or tender (or possibly all three). But fear not—this initial discomfort will likely subside after a few weeks as her body adjusts. Just be mindful. Even a simple hug could earn you a sock to the jaw.

Don't think morning sickness is limited to mornings. Nausea can strike at any time, and certain smells can trigger it—from spicy foods to caffeine to your Big Mac breath. Mom's job is to let you know what makes her feel ill; your job is to listen and keep it out of the house. Encourage her to eat smaller portions every one to two hours and not go too long on an empty stomach (per the Mayo Clinic). Mom might also have

KNOW YOUR HORMONES

Estrogen
What it does
Increases blood flow; triggers baby's organs to develop
Side effects
Tender breasts; frequent urination; pregnancy glow (!)

hCG: Human chorionic gonadotropin hormone
What it does
Suppresses Mom's immune system in case her body rejects the baby growing inside her; stimulates progesterone production
Side effects
Heightened sense of smell; morning sickness/nausea; Mom is more likely to get a cold

Progesterone
What it does
Thickens the lining of the uterine wall; prevents Mom's uterus from contracting until full term; halts menstruation
Side effects
Fatigue; heartburn; indigestion; mood swings

certain food cravings, in which case you should oblige (so long as nothing's on the off-limits list on pg. 22).

Both morning sickness and an increased need to urinate are reasons a solid dad knows where the nearest public bathroom is at all times. (This skill will serve you well when traveling with baby in the future. Hone it now.) Because she'll be peeing all the time, you should help ensure Mom stays hydrated. Buy two 40-oz bottles: one for you and one for her. Proper water intake will better your life in ways you can't possibly imagine. Resist the urge to make Edward Fortyhands jokes.

Beware of heartburn, constipation and fatigue (thanks, hormonal changes). Make sure Mom gets the rest she needs, because growing a human being is HARD WORK. Naps are encouraged. Feel free to join. Unless she says no, in which case you should leave the room and watch her sleep through a crack in the door like you're the husband in a Lifetime movie.*

Overall, the first trimester is an exciting time for both you and Mom, so take it one day at a time and try to enjoy it while it lasts.

QUESTIONS FOR YOUR DOCTOR: FIRST TRIMESTER

Beyond asking how your baby's doing, you might be curious about the following:

1. How frequently should Mom be running to the bathroom?
2. Mom's definitely been feeling nauseous. How much vomiting is *too much* vomiting?
3. Considering Mom's health and family history, is she at risk for anything? If so, what?
4. We can still have sex, right? If not, what are the factors that indicate why doing so would be unsafe or otherwise harmful to the pregnancy?
5. Can Mom still have spicy food, or is that something she ought to avoid? Why?

MYTHS BUSTED

"My mom said my partner can't be around cats while she's pregnant or it will hurt the baby!"
Not true! Interacting with cats won't increase Mom's risk of contracting toxoplasmosis, an infection that affects unborn babies. That said, the safe thing to do here is for YOU to clean the litter box while she's pregnant.

"I heard if we dangle a wedding ring on a string in front of Mom's stomach, the way it rotates will reveal the gender of the baby."
Nope, but an ultrasound will!

*Do not do this.

MORNING SICKNESS

If Mom gets sick, you better get ready to tidy up at a moment's notice. Be on alert for triggering smells. By the time baby arrives, you'll be a cleaning pro.

SEX DRIVE

Whether her libido spikes or flatlines—which, for the record, Mom has no control over—Dad should a) try not to take it personally and b) help Mom any way he can.

MOOD SWINGS

ALL of the feelings, sometimes all at once! Check in on how Mom's doing. You don't have to talk or solve all the problems. Unless she tells you to try.

CRAVINGS

Whatever Mom wants, Mom gets—in moderation. For bonus points, use this as an opportunity to be her personal chef and get creative in the kitchen.

FREQUENT URINATION

Always know where the bathroom is and make sure everyone gets plenty of water throughout the day, not just for your growing baby but for your health and sanity.

SORE BOOBS

Painful breasts suck, but it doesn't last forever. Try giving Mom a warm compress for quick relief if needed and just be mindful of their sensitivity during this time.

How to Give a Perfect Manicure

One way to help Mom feel the love throughout her pregnancy is with a bit of pampering. One easy way to do that is by treating her to a spa day at home, starting with a manicure. Set the scene by playing soothing, relaxing music and make sure she's wearing something comfortable, like a fluffy robe, which will make the second part of this spa day that much easier (see pg. 38). Don't worry if your first try out of the gate isn't top-notch. You'll get better over time.

WHAT YOU'LL NEED

These tools will help you give a professional manicure from start to finish.

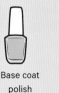

Warm bowl of water	Nail clippers	Emory board
Base coat polish	Nail Polish	Cuticle pusher

1

2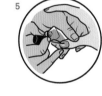

3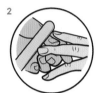

4

5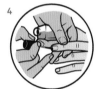

6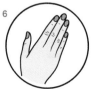

Step 1

Start by having Mom soak her hands in a bowl of warm, soapy water for five minutes. This will soften the cuticles and relax the muscles.

Step 2

Dry Mom's hands and nails with a towel, then gently push back her cuticles using a cuticle stick or a nail file. Then use the file to shape her nails by filing each finger in one direction to ensure her nail tips are either rounded or square, depending on her preference.

Step 3

Using her favorite hand lotion, lightly massage her fingers and palms. Feel free to go all out and put warm stones under her hands to rest on afterward. (Just run the stones under hot water first, then pat dry before using.)

Step 4

Wipe Mom's hands off with a towel and make sure her hands are clear of any lotion residue. Apply a thin layer of base coat to each of her nails. No need to wait—it should dry in less than a minute.

Step 5

Take Mom's favorite nail polish and apply the first (thin) coat of color across each nail using slow, even brush strokes (one to three strokes are ideal, depending on the nail). Wait two minutes to let dry.

Step 6

Apply a second coat of color to Mom's nails. Wait another two minutes before applying a thin layer of topcoat to lock in your hard work. Wait another 10 minutes or until dry to the touch, or you risk ruining all your hard work.

KNOW YOUR FLOWERS

If you want to surprise your partner (always a good idea) but don't know much about her favorite floral varieties, these petals are a pleasing place to start. A "just because" bouquet can go a long way in making Mom feel appreciated.

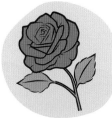

Roses
A dozen of these classics
always fits the bill.

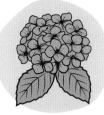

Hydrangea
Blue, pink or white,
these petals pop.

Sunflowers
Vibrant, bold and sure
to brighten her day.

Daisies
The simple, fresh,
minimalist choice.

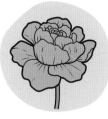

Peonies
Fluffy, fragrant
and unexpected.

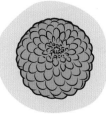

Dahlias
Over-the-top
yet elegant.

How to Give a Perfect Massage

Feel free to get creative with where you start and end and all the places in between, but if you're looking for a proper order, here's a foolproof guide to pure relaxation.

(1)

Set the mood

Play soothing music, light a candle and turn the lights low. Have plenty of towels on hand, choose some natural oils or lotions to have nearby and, for an added bonus, a warm damp towel across the eyes is a great place to start.

(4)

Spend time on the feet

Start massaging the soles by wrapping both hands around the foot and applying pressure with your thumbs. Pay special attention to the arches, as they tend to accumulate a lot of tension, but also massage the heel and the ball of the foot. When you get to the toes, give each one a gentle pull to release tension.

(5)

Work up the legs

When you're done with the feet, move onto the back of the legs. Give each leg a couple of long, relaxing strokes, all the way from the calf to the upper thigh.

② Neck, shoulders and back

Place a hand on either shoulder and knead the thumbs deep into the muscles of the shoulders and along the spine. To work on the knots, use a thumb to press around the problem area.

③ Arms and hands

Using your thumbs, massage each palm using small circular motions. Then, take each finger and slowly slide from the knuckles to the nail. Pull each finger firmly, but not so hard that you cause it to crack! Next, gently knead the arms, working up to the shoulders.

❸

HAVE SOME FUN!

There's no reason that the massage needs to be professional. Take this opportunity to explore your partner's body and maybe both of you will enjoy the moment.

❻

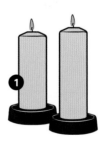

❶

If Mom isn't comfortable laying on her stomach, you can place a wedge under one of her hips to shift her uterus to the side.

⑥ End with the head

Ask your partner to flip over, then use your thumbs to massage the scalp. Now, press the center of the forehead with your fingertips. Release. Repeat for 30 seconds. Massage temples in slow circular motions.

How to Lose the Dad Bod...
By What You Eat

If you have an unhealthy diet, there's no better time to change it than right now. Not to dumb things down too much, but you want to eat as many vegetables as possible and limit foods high in fat, cholesterol and sugar.

If you're someone who likes a good tip list, here are nine simple practices that'll help you shed unwanted body weight.

Remember
Healthy eating is a lifestyle choice. Fad diets or pills won't get you lasting results.

1
Base your meals on higher fiber starchy carbohydrates like brown rice and whole wheat pasta.

2
Eat more fish, including a portion of oily fish like salmon or trout a week.

3
Eat less salt.

4
HYDRATE. Drink 6–8 glasses of water a day.

5
Don't skip breakfast.

6
Increase your protein intake.

7
Bake or roast your food instead of frying.

8
Avoid sugary beverages (including booze).

9
Everything (again, including booze) in moderation.

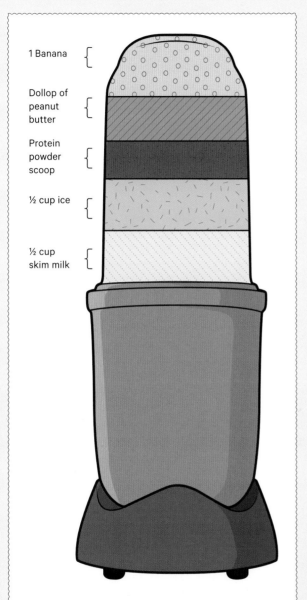

1 Banana

Dollop of peanut butter

Protein powder scoop

½ cup ice

½ cup skim milk

Invest in a mini blender Great for protein shakes and single serving purees.

THINGS TO AVOID...

White bread
Beer
Fats
Fast food
Butter
Sugar
Pasta
Excess sodium
Ice cream
Pizza
Cheese
Lunch meat
Mayonnaise
Candy
Chips
Fried food
BBQ sauce
Soft drinks
Cake

...AND TO OMIT FROM YOUR LIFE ENTIRELY

Smoking
Stress
All-nighters
Sitting for long periods
Negativity
Violence
Bad vibes

EMBRACE THE PROTEIN SHAKE

Making your own protein shake is a good way to limit your intake of carbohydrates and increase your protein. Blend the ingredients listed above for a quick, delicious and healthy snack.

Chapter 2

MONTHS THREE THROUGH SIX

→ Mom is still going through a lot of physical changes, so as Dad, you need to be prepared for baby's arrival. From showers to strollers, your journey into being Dad continues.

The Announcement

Mom will start to show around 15 weeks, after which folks will likely start to ask if the reason Mom isn't drinking is because she's trying to lose weight. You may want to head those queries off at the pass by planning the announcement that yes, this is really happening.

Thirteen weeks is a nice round number in terms of waiting, and has the benefit of falling after the first ultrasound, which means you can (and should) feel a little more secure in sharing the exciting news. But in terms of how you feel, it all comes down to how comfortable you and Mom are about sharing how dramatically your lives are about to change.

As far as how to tell your friends and loved ones, technology has provided us with more ways to do that than anyone could ever need.

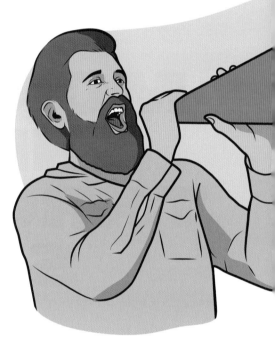

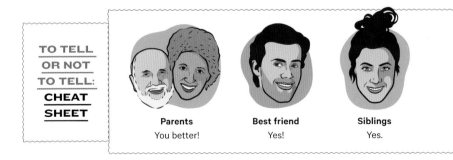

TO TELL OR NOT TO TELL: CHEAT SHEET

Parents
You better!

Best friend
Yes!

Siblings
Yes.

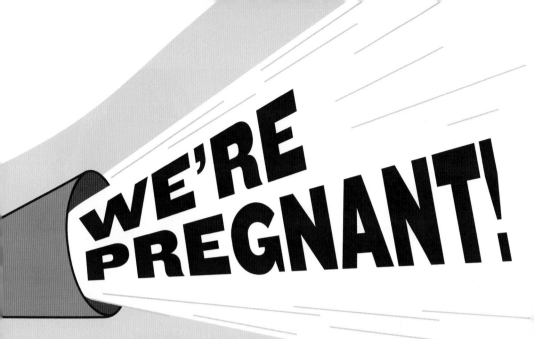

WE'RE PREGNANT!

To Tweet
or Not to Tweet

Whether you set up a Zoom room, craft a thoughtful post or shoot off a few texts, you should still call or visit your parents if you're able (and formally let HR know you might be taking some time off in a few months). Use a hashtag to organize responses and add even more personality. Be prepared to hear from people you haven't spoken to since middle school congratulating you.

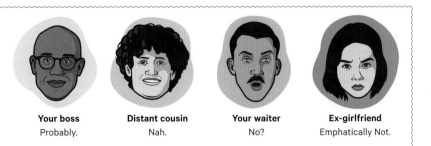

Your boss
Probably.

Distant cousin
Nah.

Your waiter
No?

Ex-girlfriend
Emphatically Not.

The Registry

This might just be one of the most fun activities you and Mom can do prior to welcoming your baby: pick out all the things you could possibly need to welcome your baby home (and some stuff just for you), and then your loved ones go and get them for you ("It takes a village," etc.). Here are some of the items you'll want to put on your registry.

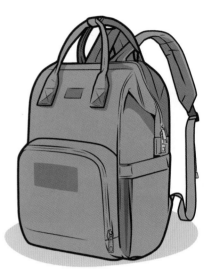

Diaper bag
This holds pacifiers, diapers, a changing pad, clothes (even a spare tee for you), snacks, bottles and more.

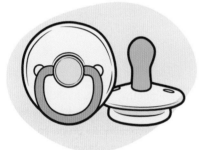

Pacifiers
Build up a stockpile so you're never without. Should your baby develop a preference, make sure to buy extras. They have a way of vanishing inexplicably.

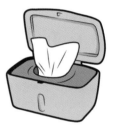

Baby wipe dispenser with weighted plate
The weight that holds the wipes in place is essential for a fast diaper change with little fuss.

MAKE IT A DATE!

Shopping for your registry can be a fun date night for Mom and Dad. Download a registry app or use the in-store scanners to keep track of everything you like, then share your registry with friends and family.

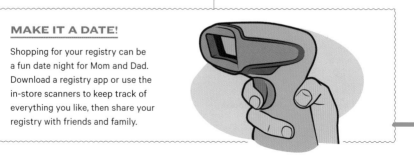

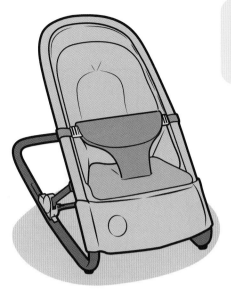

DAD HACK
Register in more than one store and have a variety of high- to low-priced items so gifting can be made easy on any budget.

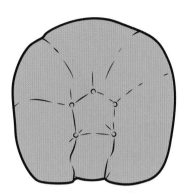

Baby bouncer

When your baby is 3 to 6 months old, the bouncer (aka jumper) will help them develop their leg strength.

Baby pillow

A great hands-free place for your baby to lounge comfortably in a propped up position (just be sure to keep them supervised).

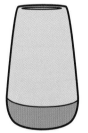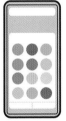

Noisemaker

Be it a modern noisemaker controlled by your phone or just a classic white noise machine, you'll want one.

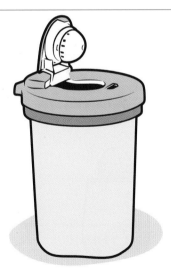

Sippy cups

You don't need these right away, but you will soon. And you'll want more than you have.

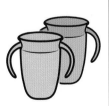

Diaper pail

This device keeps messes and smells to a minimum when you dispose of diapers. Not aesthetically pleasing, but functional.

The Registry
(CONTINUED)

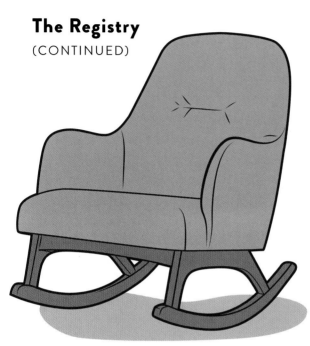

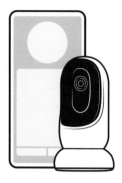

Baby monitor
High-tech moms and dads will appreciate the convenience of Wi-Fi–connected cameras (with audio!) so you can check on your baby while you're Neflix-and-chilling in another room.

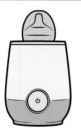

Rocking chair
Try out an array of models to see what feels right for both of you. Lighter colors show stains more easily (note: there will be stains) so darker colors mean lower maintenance.

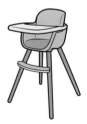

High chair
If you have the room for some items you will definitely be needing in the future, the registry is a great time to get a quality high chair.

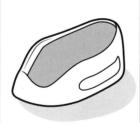

Bottle warmer
There are a lot of ways to warm up a bottle, but this makes it easy for late-night feedings.

Baby bathtub
No need to plop your newborn into the kitchen sink—use this instead.

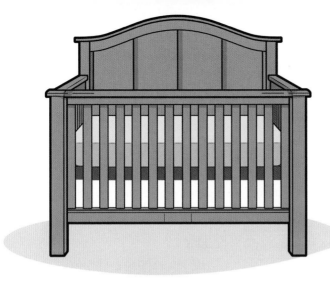

Crib

This is a big ticket item that gives people an opportunity to go in together. See more crib details on pg. 56.

Mattress

These are sold separately, so make sure to register for one and make sure it fits the crib frame exactly!

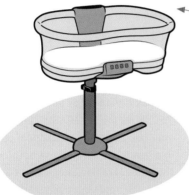

Bassinet

For the first few months, you're going to put the baby in one of these close to the bed so you can attend to their needs without having to leave the room.

A NOTE ABOUT BIG TICKET ITEMS

Babies are expensive, and you've already got a lot on your plate. This is the time to let your village help you out. Do the research and ask around, then build your registry around the high-quality items you find. You'll be surprised how many folks come through for you. At the very least, you'll keep returned items to a minimum.

DIAPERS

Whether you prefer disposable or the eco-friendly cloth variety, you'll need as many of these as you can get—and in different sizes.

Baby Clothes

Even though they are the least objectionable of all naked humans, your baby is going to need some clothes, and their sartorial situation changes as they age. Here's what to look for.

1. 0–3 Months clothes

Your baby will outgrow newborn clothes long before you forget the sight of them exiting the birth canal. Stick with buying 0–3 months clothes, which are just large enough to accommodate your growing baby without constricting their limbs in an unsafe way.

2. Cotton mitts

You won't realize this in the halcyon days of your pre-parental haze, but your baby has super sharp fingernails. Make sure they don't injure themselves (or you) by stocking up on lightweight, breathable mittens, which are also designed for wear during sleep.

3. Caps or hats

Baby's head is gonna look weird for a few months. Keep them warm and spare them the embarrassment by investing in a soft breathable cap. If you plan on taking your baby outside, look for a brimmed hat that will protect their sensitive skin from the sun.

4. Bibs

These are going to get messy multiple times a day, so find some that are easy to clean rather than cute for cute's sake. (That's a solid rule for any baby item, really. Most are cute by default.)

5. Socks, slippers or booties

Yes, shoes are ADORABLE, but your baby's going to kick them off in a heartbeat if they don't outgrow them first. Frankly, shoes aren't a necessity until your child starts walking. Stick with socks if you're staying home, but if there's a chill in the air and you're about to go out, warm slippers and booties should do the trick.

TOWELS WITH HOODS
Look, you're in too deep, pal—this is peak functionality meets ultimate cuteness. Especially the ones that make your child look like a tiny dinosaur.

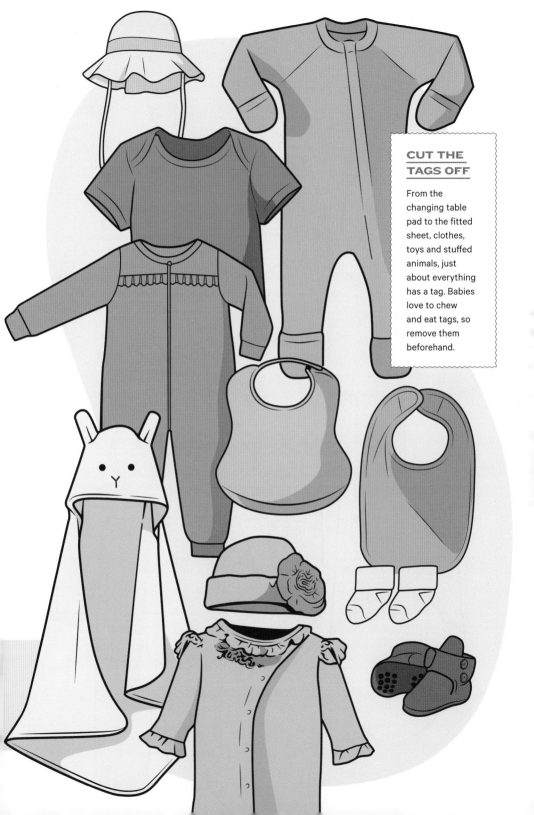

CUT THE TAGS OFF

From the changing table pad to the fitted sheet, clothes, toys and stuffed animals, just about everything has a tag. Babies love to chew and eat tags, so remove them beforehand.

BUNDLE UP!

Determine how old your baby will be when they experience their first autumn and winter and buy their seasonal wear accordingly to keep them warm and snug.

Different Types of Baby Clothes

A little knowledge goes a long way when it comes to prepping for your little one's comfort and freedom of movement.

1. Swaddles

Swaddling helps your baby feel cozy and warm while preventing them from flailing their arms or legs during sleep (in other words, swaddles help you sleep through the night, too). Not all babies like being wrapped like a burrito in a breathable blanket, though, so no sweat if your little one prefers other pajamas. AS ALWAYS, MAKE SURE YOU PLACE BABY TO SLEEP ON THEIR BACK—more on that later.

2. Bodysuits, footies, sleepers, sleep n' plays

Whether you love or hate the cutesy nomenclature, these are all essentially the same thing: footed full-body clothing your baby can wear all day, sleep in at night or (blessedly) sleep in during the day. You're going to want to stick with zippers or magnets for these as opposed to snaps, which are no one's friend when you need to change a diaper close to nap time or in the middle of the night. If you're eyeing your baby and getting jealous of their cozy, comfy duds, invest in a Kigurumi for yourself. No judgment.

3. Onesies & coveralls

Imagine the bodysuits, footies, etc. from before but without the leg or feet portion of the material and boom, you've got onesies and coveralls. Again, save future you and Mom the trouble and steer clear of anything with snaps.

4. Other tips:

✓ Wash everything BEFORE your baby wears it.

✓ Remember to grab winter coats, swimsuits and other seasonal options.

✓ Stocking up on clothes that have built-in mittens means the sleep-deprived you won't have to worry about misplacing accessories.

✓ Have lots of muslin burp cloths (aka rags for them to spit up on) ready to grab at a moment's notice.

The Nursery Theme

Designing a nursery can be a fun project for Mom and Dad to do together, and it starts by picking a theme. To get the ball rolling, here's a creative idea board to share with Mom and start brainstorming.

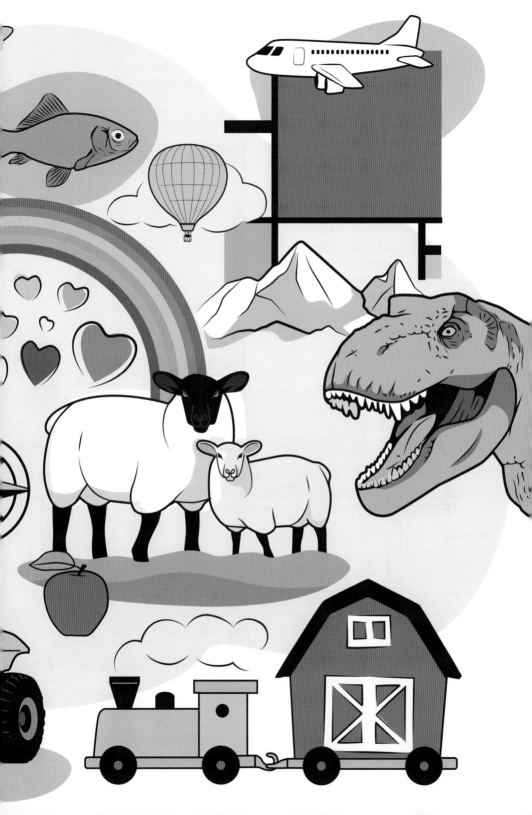

The Nursery

Once you've chosen the theme (Soothing? Exciting? Minimalist? Whatever's on clearance?), plan what major items will need to fit where—the crib, the changing station and a rocking or gliding chair—and build out from their positions in the room. The goal is to have easy access to what your baby needs and maximum comfort for you and Mom.

Window blinds
Darken a room at any time of day. Install blackout curtains if the nursery is too bright.

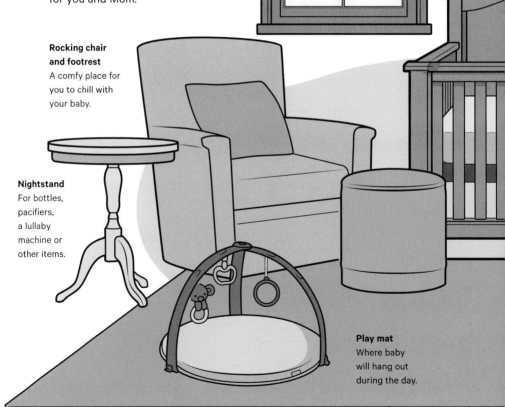

Rocking chair and footrest
A comfy place for you to chill with your baby.

Nightstand
For bottles, pacifiers, a lullaby machine or other items.

Play mat
Where baby will hang out during the day.

Baby monitor
Place this over or near the crib and then check the angle for optimal viewing.

Mobile
Great way to showcase your nursery theme while keeping it just out of baby's reach. Hang it above the crib and ensure it's secure. Choosing a high contrast mobile can make it easier for baby to enjoy.

SAFETY FIRST

1. Opt for cordless shades.
2. Choose standing lamps with a wide base for added stability.
3. Employ outlet covers for all electrical outlets.
4. Install baby gates and guards on windows and doors (they won't pose much of an issue until baby starts crawling).

Lamp
For late night diaper changes. Don't put this too close to the crib or changing table, though—it's bright.

Minimize
Any extra "things" are best kept to a minimum.

Changing table
See pg. 58 for more details.

Carpet
An area rug makes the room more comfortable.

AIR PURIFIER
An essential item to keep dust, pet dander and weird baby smells at bay.

Diaper bin
Position this close to the changing table.

Preparing the Changing Table

You can't clean a mess with a mess. Just like a chef adheres to the practice of mise en place ("everything in its place") before preparing a delicious meal, you'll want to have your changing table set up before dealing with the wholly unappetizing creation your

bundle of joy has been roasting in its diaper. Baby wipes, diapers, petroleum jelly and a diaper pail are all essentials you'll want to have handy at all times. You can keep the station clean and ready-to-use by storing the less commonly needed items in the top drawers.

(1)

Diapers
About a dozen(ish) should do the trick.

(2)

Petroleum jelly
You're gonna wanna use this generously.

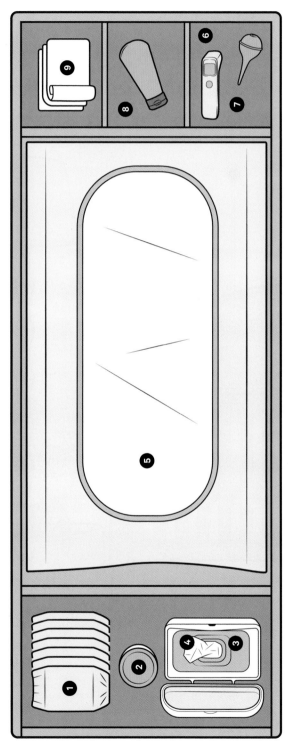

③

Weighted baby wipe dispenser

Notice the "weighted"—this is important for those one-handed grabs you'll get really good at.

④

Unscented, water-based wipes

These will clean your baby while keeping the environment clean, too.

⑤

Changing pad and cover

These are sold separately from the changing table, believe it or not (don't learn this the hard way). You want one.

⑥

Thermometer

Rectal thermometers are best for babies. Storing with the changing table prevents unfortunate mix-ups with your personal oral version.

⑦

Nasal suction

Clears out congestion as needed.

⑧

Lotion

Keep the little one well-moisturized.

⑨

Extra pads, burp rags

Spit-up happens. Be ready.

⑩

Drawers

Extra diapers, trash bags and baby wipes—keep close by but out of the way.

SET UP A CHANGING TABLE DOWNSTAIRS

Do yourself a favor: If you live in a two-story home, set up a downstairs changing station. This can be a pared down version of your nursery table, or a blanket that you toss on a countertop or dining table for quick changes that'll rival the best of Broadway.

How to Pick a Bottle and Keep It Clean

Picking out the right baby bottle for your child can be a tough and somewhat boring decision. Try several and see what the little tyke prefers. Basically, you want to minimize the amount of air they swallow. Gulping air causes gas and discomfort, which no one wants at mealtime.

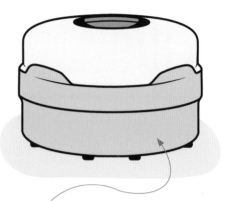

Bottle sanitizer and bottle brush
The one-two punch in bottle cleaning

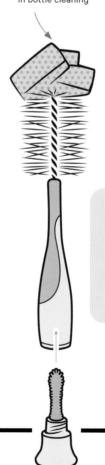

Foam tip
Sponge area that is gentle and adaptable

Bristles
Great for removing excess buildup

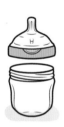

Wide nipple surface
Easy to clean and imitates a breast

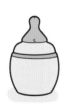

Plastic bottle
Lots of options to choose from and very affordable

SOAP + WATER
Along with your cleaning tools, soap and water should be your go-to cleaning utilities.

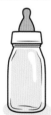

Glass bottle
Doesn't absorb colors and is dishwasher safe

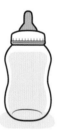

Silicone
Imitates skin and easy for baby to hold

Firm tip
Most brushes have a hidden nipple brush in the handle for tough to clean spots

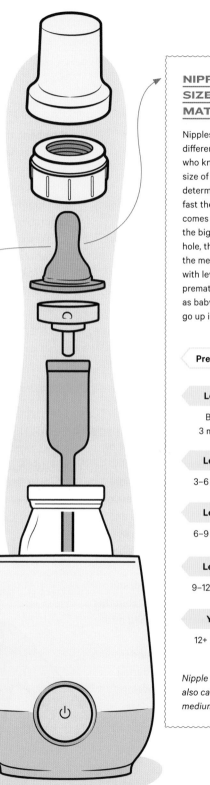

Bottle cap
Essential if you're
on the move or
traveling

Nipple ring
Holds nipple and
any other bottle
components
in place

Nipple
See chart
to the right

Venting system
Many baby bottle
have some form
of venting system
that is good for
gas reduction
and colic.

Bottle
Milk or
formula here

Bottle warmer
If Mom is pumping
and freezing her
milk, a bottle
warmer is very
handy.

NIPPLE SIZE MATTERS!

Nipples come in
different sizes,
who knew?! The
size of the hole
determines how
fast the liquid
comes out, so
the bigger the
hole, the faster
the meal. Start
with level 1 (or
premature) and
as baby grows,
go up in size.

Premature

Level 1
Birth–
3 months

Level 2
3–6 Months

Level 3
6–9 Months

Level 4
9–12 Months

Y-cut
12+ Months

*Nipple sizes are
also called slow,
medium, and fast*

Second Trimester Ailments and Solutions

The second trimester of pregnancy, roughly week 14 through 27 (aka the "Yes this is legitimately happening" phase), is the time when your baby truly begins to take shape. Here's what to expect.

Whether or not you've announced the happy news to friends and family, congratulations are in order because many moms consider this trimester to be the most pleasant of the three. Mom's body is becoming more acclimated to the new human being growing inside her—the worst of the morning sickness is usually gone, she's starting to feel more like herself again (albeit a version of herself that's doubling as an incubator) and your baby is still small enough to not cause Mom too much discomfort.

Another bonus: You, Dad, still have time to get your sh*t together before welcoming your child into the world.

Your growing baby is undergoing some amazing changes during this time. Their lungs develop; their fingernails, fingerprints and footprints form; not only can they hear, they can also begin to recognize your voice among other exciting milestones. By the end of the second trimester, your baby will be roughly as long as a zucchini (adorable!).

Likewise, Mom's body isn't anywhere close to done changing and growing, most notably her belly and breasts. If she hasn't already begun showing, Mom will start to have a bump during this

> "The second trimester was great. All the adverse symptoms were gone...and my energy was back."
> —ELYSE G.

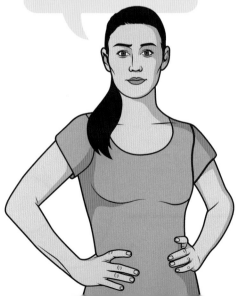

HOW TO MANAGE STRETCH MARKS

There's no one surefire way to prevent stretch marks, but you can do your Dad-ly duty and help Mom follow these tips if she would rather keep them at a minimum.

Step 1: Stay hydrated

An increased H2O intake will help boost the elasticity of Mom's skin, making it less prone to tearing.

Step 2: Load up on vitamins

If you've been following the What to Eat section (pg. 20), you're off to a great start. Focus on foods that are high in vitamin A, vitamin E, antioxidants and omega-3s, all of which nourish and protect skin.

Step 3: Get moving

Stretching and light cardio are the goal. Mom should consult her doctor about which exercises (if any) are best for her.

Step 4: Watch your weight

It's a given that Mom's going to gain weight during pregnancy (and it's a good thing!), but gaining a great deal of weight in a short amount of time could put undue stress on her skin, making it more likely to tear. Mom's doctor can weigh in on healthy target weight ranges.

Step 5: Use moisturizer

Don't worry about splurging on expensive creams (unless Mom's all about that)—look for a lotion that has ingredients like collagen and shea butter. Read the labels carefully and avoid anything with retinols or retinoids in the ingredients.

time and will likely transition to wearing super comfortable and stretchy maternity clothes full-time. She might also have more of an appetite now. Tip: You might consider shooting a week-by-week or month-by-month photo session of Mom to document the process and save it for your baby's first photo album. Or turn it into a slideshow for the baby shower!

Week 20 marks the halfway point of Mom's pregnancy (or 18 weeks after conception, if you want to get technical). This also might be when Mom feels the baby move for the first time—that fluttering-in-her-stomach feeling—which is called quickening.

All of this growing and changing (for Mom) means she's going to experience some skin issues: the hormones coursing through her body, for one, can prompt dark patches of skin to appear on her face (melasma). A dark vertical line (called linea nigra) might also show up spanning the length of her abdomen. Mom's producing more melanin in her body right now—you can mostly thank the estrogen for that—but these marks usually disappear after she delivers the baby. Wearing sunscreen will help prevent the marks from darkening.

Other things Mom might experience during this time due to surging hormones or changes in circulation include congestion, constipation, dizziness, heartburn, leg cramps, sensitive gums while brushing or flossing, urinary tract infections, vaginal discharge, and Braxton Hicks contractions.

In terms of hormones, Mom's still got estrogen and progesterone coursing through her veins. Her ovaries will also produce relaxin, which keeps the cervix and uterus relaxed (hence the name) and also helps the placenta to grow. It might also cause Mom to feel more aches and discomfort in her ligaments.

Cortisol increases during this time, and while you might already know it as the stress hormone, during pregnancy, cortisol helps

regulate blood sugar levels and manage Mom's metabolism. Too much cortisol, though, might be linked to blood pressure ailments and possibly stretch marks.

There's also a hormone that's produced by the pituitary gland: prolactin, which preps Mom's milk glands for breastfeeding and causes her breasts to grow.

QUESTIONS FOR YOUR DOCTOR: SECOND TRIMESTER

Beyond asking how your baby's doing, you might be curious about the following:

1. What symptoms are normal? Abnormal?
2. What are some potential complications we might face?
3. Should Mom have already started sleeping on her side? Is sleeping on her back safe?
4. What kinds of exercise are safe at this stage?
5. Is spotting normal or will it always send us into a spiral of doom?
6. How can we better manage Mom's discomfort? What medications can she take right now?

MYTHS BUSTED:

Girl babies arrive early and boys arrive late.
False! The baby's sex does not factor into when labor begins.

BRAXTON HICKS CONTRACTIONS

When muscles in Mom's uterus tighten in an uncomfortable and nonrhythmic way for 30 to 60 seconds at a time after certain activities like sex or other exercise or when she's dehydrated. This is NORMAL, but call your doctor if they worsen over time.

DIZZINESS

To combat this feeling, Mom should drink lots of fluids, not stand for long periods of time, stand up slowly if sitting down or simply lie down and rest.

HEMORRHOIDS

These can come part and parcel with constipation and straining during bowel movements. A soothing warm bath should help relieve any discomfort, as should applying ice packs. For more relief, Mom's doctor can prescribe or recommend pregnancy-safe medicines (e.g., stool softeners).

LEG CRAMPS

To avoid them, Mom should stay hydrated as well as stretch before bed, take a warm bath or use an ice pack, wear supportive shoes or ask her doctor for a magnesium supplement.

VAGINAL DISCHARGE

If Mom's wetness has a strong odor, strange color or comes with an itching or burning sensation, it could be a sign of a vaginal infection—if so, Mom should see her doctor ASAP.

VARICOSE VEINS

These unsightly blue, twisted-looking veins should improve somewhat after Mom gives birth. Mom shouldn't stand or sit for long periods. While lying down or sitting, she should keep her feet propped up like the proper queen she is.

Strolling Into Dad Life

Get ready for one of the most impactful decisions you'll make as a soon-to-be dad: stroller choice. You don't want to be the one knocking your baby awake on a dirt trail because you went for the city slicker stroller, nor do you want to be the owner of the unwieldy country carriage when navigating through a crowded restaurant. Knowing what your needs are is key to making the right choice.

PRACTICE!
Once you've chosen a stroller, practice folding and unfolding it before the baby arrives so that when it's actually in use you'll be an old pro.

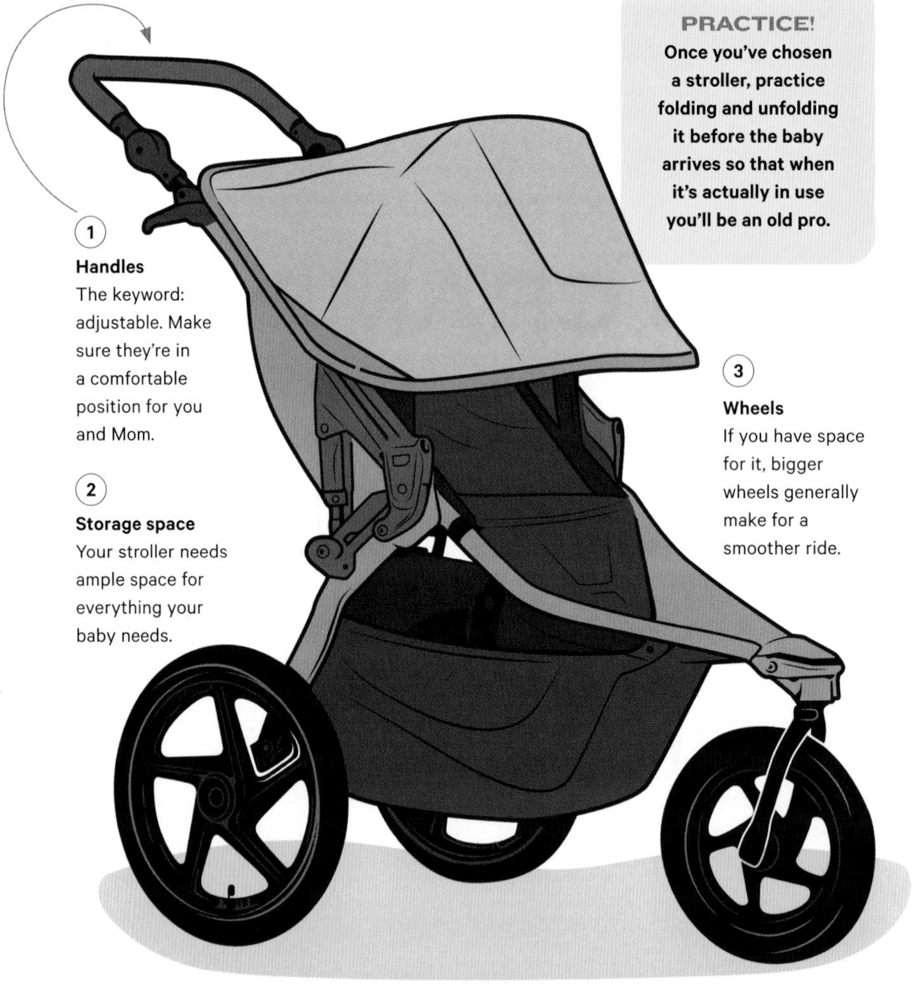

1

Handles
The keyword: adjustable. Make sure they're in a comfortable position for you and Mom.

2

Storage space
Your stroller needs ample space for everything your baby needs.

3

Wheels
If you have space for it, bigger wheels generally make for a smoother ride.

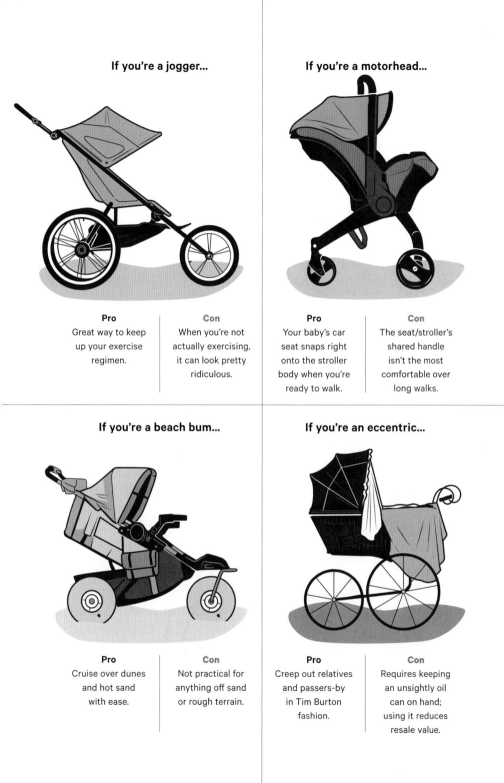

If you're a jogger...

Pro
Great way to keep up your exercise regimen.

Con
When you're not actually exercising, it can look pretty ridiculous.

If you're a motorhead...

Pro
Your baby's car seat snaps right onto the stroller body when you're ready to walk.

Con
The seat/stroller's shared handle isn't the most comfortable over long walks.

If you're a beach bum...

Pro
Cruise over dunes and hot sand with ease.

Con
Not practical for anything off sand or rough terrain.

If you're an eccentric...

Pro
Creep out relatives and passers-by in Tim Burton fashion.

Con
Requires keeping an unsightly oil can on hand; using it reduces resale value.

How to Lose the Dad Bod...
By What You Do

Whether you already have a dad bod or you're hoping to avoid one, it's about to get a lot harder to find the time to keep this meme-worthy fatherly physique at bay. But it's not at all impossible. You just have to focus on diet, exercise and the determination to commit to both equally. If you don't already have some, start by investing in a couple of dumbbells (15 lb is a good starting point).

To get yourself moving in the right direction, try adding a few things to your weekly routine that will help shed extra pounds and add some definition.

1

Cardio
Try running for 30 minutes or biking for 40 minutes. Cardio is essential for losing weight, so get moving!

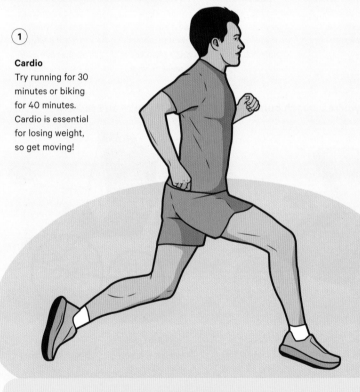

DISCLAIMER
While these exercises can work wonders for many dads, be sure to check with your doctor before starting any new fitness program.

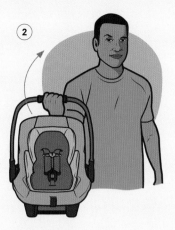

Car seat curls

This bicep booster will prepare you to frequently carry the car seat to and from vehicles. With a dumbbell gripped underhand in each hand, stand with your feet shoulder width apart and your knees slightly bent. Keeping your elbows pointed at your hips, curl the dumbbells upward, squeezing your biceps. Straighten your arms back out and repeat.

Diaper bag curls

Normally known as hammer curls, these will help you get used to the motion of putting that diaper bag on your shoulder. With your palms facing inward and thumbs facing up, hold the weights at your sides. Keeping your elbows pulled into your sides, curl the weights up to your shoulders. Slowly extend your arms down and repeat as you're able.

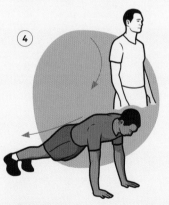

Burpees

These increase strength and endurance so you can hold and burp your baby for as long as it takes. With your arms at your sides and your feet shoulder width apart, squat down and place your hands on the floor in front of you. Kick your legs back into a plank position, then quickly bring your legs forward, back into a squat. Return to the starting position, repeat.

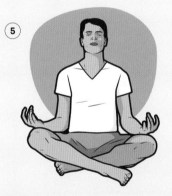

Meditation

You owe it to yourself to carve out a few minutes of calm every day. Set a timer, get in a comfortable seated position and focus on your breathing. Inhale for four counts. Hold your breath for a beat then exhale for at least four counts. Some people prefer the 4-7-8 method, but find what's comfortable for you. Repeat as necessary.

Chapter 3

MONTHS SIX THROUGH NINE

⟶ You're in a good groove, the stage is set, and now: the waiting game. These last three months of your partner's pregnancy are the perfect time to set the whole family up for success.

Baby's on the Move and Ready to Groove

One of the most exciting parts of the pregnancy will be when your partner starts to feel the telltale kicks, punches and other prenatal kung-fu moves of your future family member. Here's what you can do when the flailing begins.

Trust your partner

As always, Mom can be trusted to know certain things...well... better than you. If she notices any dramatic changes in frequency, intensity, duration or other patterns of movement, trust her observations. A 2014 Swedish study found that expecting mothers can be quite acutely attuned to these changes, which aren't necessarily a bad thing.

Encourage your baby

As any doctor will tell you, the movement you're feeling in your partner's abdomen is baby's

exercise, and that's a good thing. On the other hand, if the trend your partner is feeling is toward less movement, there are things you can do to encourage your baby to get moving. For example, if you've noticed your baby is prone to move around more at the OB-GYN's office during the ultrasound, that's because the gentle pressure and movement of the wand can perk your baby up. You can do the same thing yourself using a wand-like implement—maybe a spatula? Get creative. Just be gentle!

Don't underestimate the power

According to *Healthline*, at 30 weeks, a baby's legs can generate up to 10½ pounds of force. As the growing baby runs out of room, this figure depletes until birth, when things start to feel pretty cramped. But those baby boogie-woogies can still be pretty forceful as your little one practices their 1-inch punch.

This is yet another reason to let Mom relax as you complete the tasks that might not feel so pleasant to do while the creature in her belly reenacts the coffin escape sequence from *Kill Bill: Volume 2*.

> **IT'S TRUE!**
> The voices and music that baby hears in utero do, in fact, help them get used to their outside environment.

WHAT TO TRY AND WHAT TO AVOID WITH MOM'S NOTICEABLY PREGNANT BELLY

Make the most of this last stage of pregnancy and have a bit of fun with your partner's protuberant belly with these lighthearted activities.

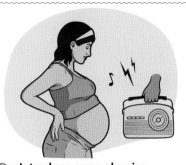

Do: Introduce some classics

Bust out everything from Mozart to Led Zeppelin to see what tracks your baby responds to most (and pray it isn't polka).

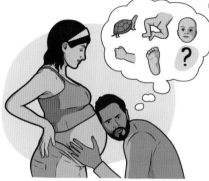

Do: Play "what is that?"

Is it a foot? A hand? Indigestion from last night's pad thai? We just don't know!

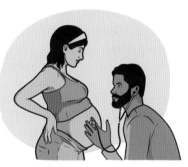

Do: Use a stethoscope

You don't need a PhD to hear what's happening in Mom's belly. Borrow a stethoscope and give it a listen!

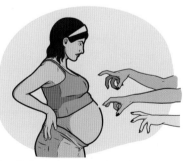

Don't: Let strangers touch without asking

Random people may (read: will) try to touch Mom's belly. It's creepy. Dad should help enforce an "always ask" policy.

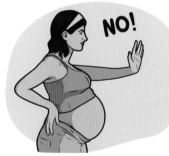

Do: Have a plan for saying no

Brainstorming replies for Mom, like, "Please don't, my skin is sensitive today," will help when what Mom really wants to do is unleash hell on would-be tummy touchers.

The Babymoon

There's no time like the present to cherish these last few weeks you'll have alone with Mom. Before it gets too close to baby's due date, carve out some quality one-on-one time and take a relaxing trip while you still know what eight uninterrupted hours of sleep feels like.

Keep in mind Mom should abstain from flying or taking long trips by car, bus or train at about 36 weeks into her pregnancy. Mom should also limit her activities to avoid anything with jarring movements—yep, that means no dune buggy joyrides, roller coasters or bungee jumping.

You won't want to venture anywhere too remote or off the beaten path in case you need to seek medical assistance in the event of an emergency.

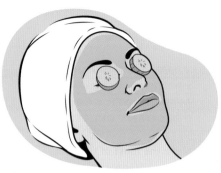

Spa getaway
Whether your wellness regimen includes an hour-long massage, facial or both, get it in while you can.

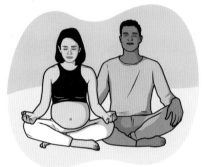

Meditation retreat
If you're looking to clear your mind and rediscover your inner peace before a tiny human requires your assistance 24/7, this will be your moment (or weekend) of zen. Namaste.

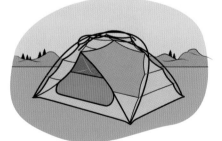

Camping
Now is not the time to scale Machu Picchu, but a low-intensity hike, weekend of camping or cabin stay might be just what the doctor ordered—so long as said doctor approves of Mom hiking.

DON'T BREAK THE BANK
There's no need to blow baby's college fund for a stay at the Ritz. But check to see if you've got miles or hotel perk points to burn (you can't pay for college with Disney Dollars, after all).

KEEP IT LOCAL

Who says you have to jet off to the Bahamas or Amalfi Coast to enjoy a quality babymoon? You can have just as much relaxation and fun by renting an oceanside cottage or lakefront lodge a short drive from home.

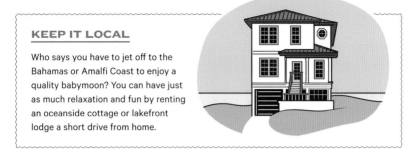

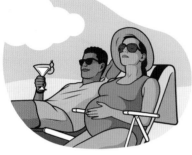

Beach trip

Pack a meal and an umbrella, then get ready to soak in that sweet sunshine and enjoy watching the tide roll in. Just be sure everyone's wearing sunscreen and staying hydrated. (Consider it practice for the future.)

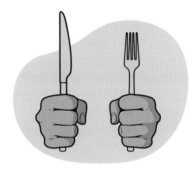

Food adventure

If you and Mom are foodies, plan a long weekend of indulgence—e.g., a guided food tour or an improvised pizza crawl—and send those taste buds on a wild ride. Build your itinerary around whatever Mom's been craving for extra Dad points.

NORTH 1 ←

SOUTH 1 →

If you're on the East Coast, driving Route 1 south is a great road trip, which can be a fun adventure without added airfare.

KEY WEST

If you've never been, now is a great time to go. Whether you decide to fly or take a long drive south (with plenty of rest stops, of course), the Florida Keys is a great place to unwind in a low-key island setting.

Nesting Is a Thing

When there's a baby on the way, it's natural to go a bit overboard when it comes to planning and prepping. For pregnant women, this instinct is colloquially referred to as nesting, and it usually entails thoroughly cleaning and reorganizing the home in the weeks leading up to the baby's birth. Nesting during pregnancy is not harmful to Mom or baby, but there are precautions you'll want to take (if only to ensure you don't bite off more than you can chew).

Dad should help with any heavy objects or furniture moving. Mom's equilibrium may be a little off, or at the very least her center of gravity is more forward than usual, so carrying anything up and down stairs should be done with great care. And if you're doing some deep cleaning, ensure you have good ventilation and avoid the use of harsh cleaning chemicals such as bleach or oven cleaners.

PRO MOVE
Add felt pads to the bottom of your furniture legs. It will protect your floors and make things easier to move.

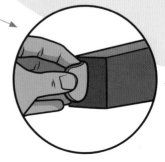

It's a good idea to have some drywall screws and anchors for decorating...and don't forget a level!

START YOUR CARE SEARCH EARLY

The last few months of pregnancy are a great time to visit daycares and interview nannies, if that's in your future. A few things to consider before you begin:

1. Location and convenience are crucial. You'll want a daycare that's close to home or a nanny who's local to make life easier.

2. Don't decide too quickly—ask for references and actually call them.

3. Anyone you entrust to care for your child should be CPR certified and trained to handle emergencies.

4. Prospective caregivers should be amenable to completing a background check, which is standard procedure for anyone in childcare.

5. Make sure the caregiving style aligns with yours or the caregiver is willing to adhere to your wishes.

6. Get to know their vaccination/ immunization policy and what happens when other children in their care are sick.

How to Nest Like a Pro

While Dad probably won't instinctively nest before the baby arrives (not that there's anything wrong with that), he can and should help Mom prepare. Here are five ways you can get involved with the male version of nesting, or "mesting" as it's unsurprisingly called in the blogosphere.

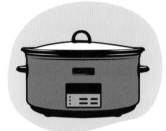

Food duty

No matter who was holding things down in the kitchen, Dad should take over cooking detail exclusively. Meal prep will free up the kitchen and keep everything clean longer. Stocking the freezer with easy-to-heat-and-eat meals (see chili, pg. 90) is a good idea as well.

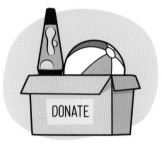

Out with the old

Sure, you could dust off and wipe down that mostly decorative minibar...or just ditch it altogether. A new baby will fill your home with accessories of all sizes in no time, so you'll want to declutter as much as you can ahead of time.

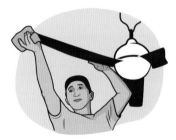

Get detailed

Now's the time to obsess over details: Is your trash can big enough for the three of you? Have you cut the tags off the baby's clothes? Is that slippery rug in the hallway a potential hazard for walking with the baby (duh)? Make a to-do list and DO it.

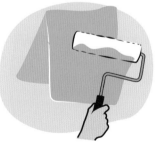

Ready the room

The nursery is your baby's "nest," so it's important to have all the fine details of this space ironed out before they arrive. Handle the painting, wallpaper or sanitizing duties beforehand so all the harmful fumes are completely aired out.

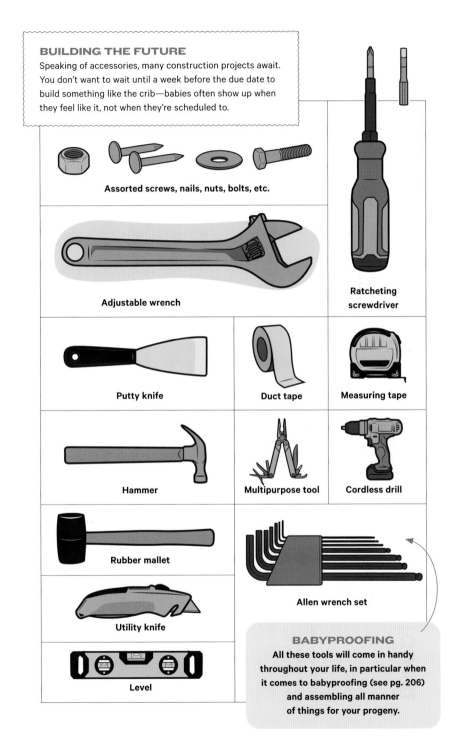

BUILDING THE FUTURE

Speaking of accessories, many construction projects await. You don't want to wait until a week before the due date to build something like the crib—babies often show up when they feel like it, not when they're scheduled to.

Assorted screws, nails, nuts, bolts, etc.

Adjustable wrench

Ratcheting screwdriver

Putty knife

Duct tape

Measuring tape

Hammer

Multipurpose tool

Cordless drill

Rubber mallet

Allen wrench set

Utility knife

Level

BABYPROOFING

All these tools will come in handy throughout your life, in particular when it comes to babyproofing (see pg. 206) and assembling all manner of things for your progeny.

The GO! Bag

While having a baby is far from the end of the world, it does share one important prep technique with the apocalypse: the trusty bug-out bag, aka GO! bag. When your partner goes into labor and it's time to head to the hospital, you shouldn't be scrambling for the essentials. Have the following items packed into your baby bug-out bag with plenty of time to spare—remember, labor can always happen early.

YOU'RE NOT MOVING IN. PACK LIGHT

The hospital should have just about everything Mom and baby will need. No need to overpack. If you do forget something, you can always have a friend or family member coordinate a drop-off.

(1)

Identification and insurance cards

Save yourself the headache and pack these first, along with copies of any relevant medical records and your birth plan.

(2)

Lip balm

For Mom, for Dad, for whoever's feeling chapped or in need of a shine.

(3)

Oral hygiene

You might be there overnight or longer, so you'll want to have toothbrushes, toothpaste and floss on hand.

(4)

Deodorant

Hospitals are stressful by default. Stress = sweat. Pack some deodorant for yourself and Mom.

(5)

Daily medications

Time doesn't stop at the hospital. If you take any prescriptions, bring them: no exceptions.

(6)

Easy snacks

Mom probably won't be allowed to eat much during your stay, but you'll want to nervously chew something other than your fingernails.

(7)

Comfy clothes

Making a good first impression matters, just not now. You'll want to be comfortable waiting for the baby, so leave the suit and tie at home.

(8)

Going home outfit (for Mom and Dad)

Things might get ugly during labor. By the time you're discharged, you'll both want a fresh set of clothes.

(9)

Going home outfit (for baby)

One is enough. Pack something fun or cute for your child's first car ride.

(10)

Thank you cards for the nurses

You're going to get real close with the nurses. A card is a simple but meaningful way to show your gratitude.

(11)

A Pen

You can't sign your child's birth certificate in Jell-O.

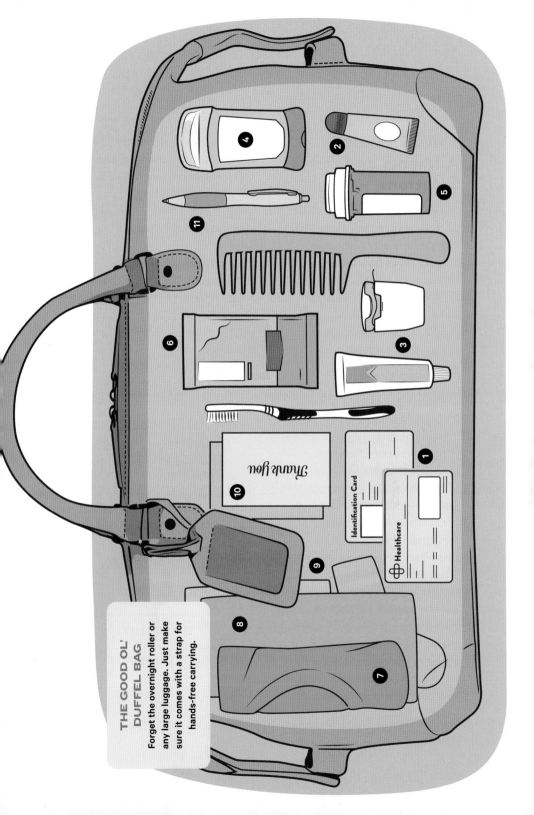

THE GOOD OL' DUFFEL BAG

Forget the overnight roller or any large luggage. Just make sure it comes with a strap for hands-free carrying.

Identification Card

✛ Healthcare

Thank you

Third Trimester Ailments and Solutions

You've finally reached that stage when Mom is not only noticeably pregnant the entire time, she also—whether from excitement, fatigue or (most likely) both— *cannot wait to have this thing already*. You might wonder at this point if Mom's been pregnant forever, and she might, too, because the woman has spent more than half a year incubating and carrying your child-to-be. Fortunately, the end is in sight!

Mom's body is in its final stages of prepping your offspring to survive outside the womb. She may or may not still be getting used to feeling the baby move their limbs or change positions suddenly throughout the day (especially when she's trying to get some sleep). But Mom's probably far too familiar with having to pee a lot, and backaches have become an everyday thing now as her body strains to accommodate her sizable stomach. She'll want to make sure her shoes have good arch support and that she isn't on her feet too long.

If it hasn't already sunk in (and it's perfectly fine if it hasn't), you're about to become a parent. This last trimester can make for a highly emotional time as you grapple with anxieties relating to your baby's health ("What if the baby comes early?"), labor plans ("What if Mom goes into labor and we're in a TGI Fridays?") and accepting your lives are about to change forever ("Do I feel parental yet?" "Am I ready for this?" "What is 'ready'—I still eat cereal with marshmallows for breakfast!"). Be sure to talk with trusted friends,

"I loved my super cute belly and watching her kick, but I also had major discomfort, like...just get this baby out!"
—GILANA B.

family members and your OB-GYN about what keeps you up at night in order to manage your fears and expectations during this time for the sake of your mental health.

Speaking of your OB-GYN: Beginning at around week 32, Mom's doctor might want her to begin coming in for more frequent checkups, which is perfectly normal albeit slightly frustrating if you don't love hanging out with medical professionals by now.

Besides making sure your child-to-be is developing on track, Mom's OB-GYN is going to focus on screening Mom for conditions such as gestational diabetes, Group B strep and iron deficiency anemia, all of which can impact your baby adversely and make life harder for Mom. Fortunately, these can be treated and managed with early intervention.

On a hormonal level, Mom's still dealing with elevated estrogen and progesterone levels, which will peak when she reaches about 32 weeks—at this point, her estrogen will be six times higher than before she was pregnant. This surge, however, also makes Mom's ankles, feet and fingers swell up. Resist the urge to call her Bloaty McBloatface.

Aside from these usual chemical

BE READY IF BABY ARRIVES EARLY

Even if you've prepped a ton, there's always a chance your baby will decide to pull a dramatic entrance by arriving earlier than anticipated. Once Mom's water breaks, it's go time, which means about a month out from the due date, you'll want to make sure you've got these critical things down pat in case things don't go according to schedule.

1. Pack your GO! bag and have it handy (see pg. 80).

2. Tell your boss (and Mom's boss) you might become a Dad in the next month or much, much sooner.

3. Acquire, sanitize and set up the items your baby and Mom will rely on immediately after you arrive back home post-delivery.

4. Arrange for someone to take care of your pet(s) while you and Mom are at the hospital. (Labor can stretch on longer than you'd imagine, and you won't want to dash back home and possibly miss your child's birth because your dog can't feed itself.)

Bonus: Ensure you understand in theory (if not in practice) how to change a diaper.

suspects, a hormone called relaxin will make its presence felt during this trimester, loosening up her ligaments and joints to get her body ready for childbirth. Unfortunately, this also makes her more prone to general aches and pains as well as wicked heartburn.

Meanwhile, another hormone, prolactin, prompts Mom's body to begin lactating. This will initially manifest as colostrum, a thick, yellowish, nutrient-rich substance leaking from her breasts that will sustain your newborn before Mom's breast milk comes in fully, after delivery. She may be dealing with a condition some medical professionals refer to as "leaky boobs." Don't make it weird.

These last months of pregnancy can drag on for what feels like an eternity—and you're not even the one carrying the baby! But there's a light at the end of the tunnel, even if your baby arrives after the due date (good luck!). Now's the

time to focus on keeping spirits up, coming to terms with your new responsibilities and cherishing your alone time while it still exists. Plan those date nights, check in with your partner and binge as much streaming content as your schedule can handle.

QUESTIONS FOR YOUR DOCTOR: THIRD TRIMESTER

Take advantage of these last few visits to ask about what to expect during labor and delivery:

1. What kinds of exercises are safe during the last trimester?
2. If I'm overdue, when should we begin discussing induction?
3. What should we do if Mom suddenly doesn't feel the baby move?
4. Is bleeding normal? How much?
5. What should we do when Mom's water breaks?
6. Where do we go when we arrive at the hospital?

MYTHS BUSTED:

Mom's water breaks in exciting fashion (maybe during a costume party!) and thus begins labor.
False—for most people, that is. This only happens with 8 to 10 percent of pregnancies. Be prepared, though.

Eating spicy foods will induce labor.
False—there are no known foods that cause labor to begin. There are some medications however...

ANXIETY

This trimester can feel like the longest, so Dad should offer Mom fun distractions or assurances. A therapist can help if you or Mom are struggling to manage your stress levels.

BLOODY SHOW

No, this isn't British slang: When the mucus plug gets dislodged, it can exit Mom's body in pieces or all at once. Yeah, there's going to be some blood involved.

HEARTBURN

This should finally go away after Mom gives birth. Until then, have antacids on hand to quell the discomfort. Eating small, frequent meals can also help.

LIGHTENING

When the baby drops/settles lower into Mom's pelvis. Whether it's a few weeks or a few hours before labor, this means Mom is inching closer to the hour of delivery.

PREGNANCY BRAIN

Stress, hormones or a lack of sleep—or all three—can make Mom feel foggy and forgetful. Start paying extra attention to what Mom needs and step in to help where you can.

SHORTNESS OF BREATH

Mom's body is under a lot of strain right now, and she might get winded more easily. Practicing proper posture can help give her lungs more room to expand.

THE WAITING GAME

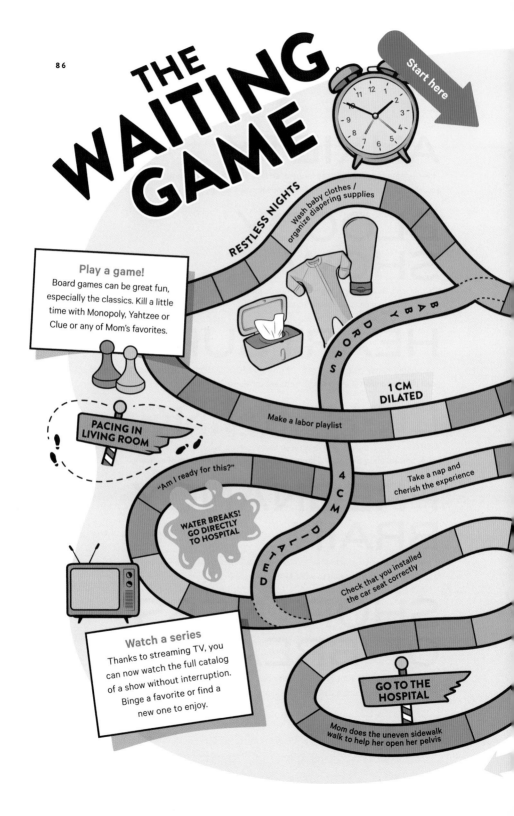

Start here

RESTLESS NIGHTS

Wash baby clothes / organize diapering supplies

BABY SPORT

Play a game!
Board games can be great fun, especially the classics. Kill a little time with Monopoly, Yahtzee or Clue or any of Mom's favorites.

1 CM DILATED

Make a labor playlist

PACING IN LIVING ROOM

"Am I ready for this?"

4 CM DILATED

Take a nap and cherish the experience

WATER BREAKS! GO DIRECTLY TO HOSPITAL

Check that you installed the car seat correctly

Watch a series
Thanks to streaming TV, you can now watch the full catalog of a show without interruption. Binge a favorite or find a new one to enjoy.

GO TO THE HOSPITAL

Mom does the uneven sidewalk walk to help her open her pelvis

You've made it! Er, almost made it. After months of excitement, planning and preparation, there's nothing left to do but watch the clock and wait for your little one to make a grand entrance. Here are some issues you might run into and a few ideas on how to survive this time with your sanity mostly intact.

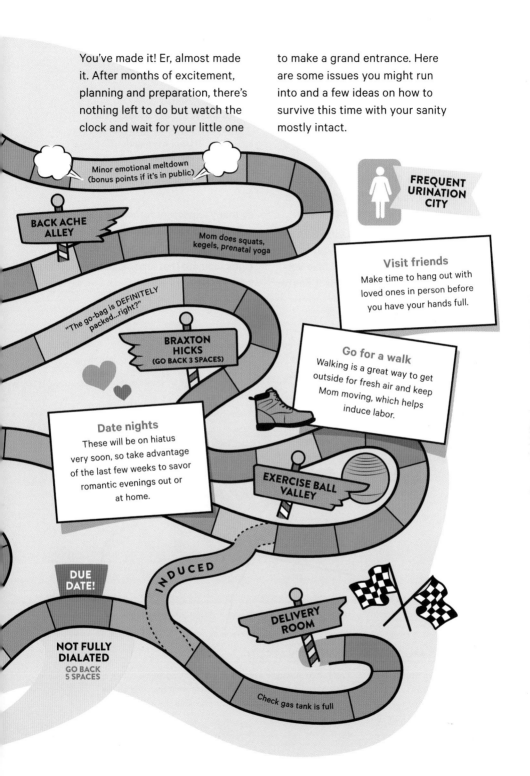

Minor emotional meltdown (bonus points if it's in public)

FREQUENT URINATION CITY

BACK ACHE ALLEY

Mom does squats, kegels, prenatal yoga

Visit friends
Make time to hang out with loved ones in person before you have your hands full.

"The go-bag is DEFINITELY packed...right?"

BRAXTON HICKS
(GO BACK 3 SPACES)

Go for a walk
Walking is a great way to get outside for fresh air and keep Mom moving, which helps induce labor.

Date nights
These will be on hiatus very soon, so take advantage of the last few weeks to savor romantic evenings out or at home.

EXERCISE BALL VALLEY

DUE DATE!

INDUCED

NOT FULLY DIALATED
GO BACK 5 SPACES

DELIVERY ROOM

Check gas tank is full

Signs That Labor Has Begun

CALL FIRST!
It's always a good idea to call your OB-GYN physician when any sign of labor has begun.

Your most valuable asset in this arena is your well-honed ability to trust your partner. Mom will tell you when it's go time, but there are some signs you can look out for so that the moment doesn't take you completely by surprise, as it has for so many expectant fathers before you. According to the Cleveland Clinic and *Healthline*, the following signs indicate that labor is between 24 and 48 hours away.

(1)

Five minutes between contractions
Start the timer when Mom says she feels "the wave" of contraction pain beginning, and stop it when the pain expires. When the time between contractions is less than five minutes, it's time to head to the hospital.

(2)

Listen to Mom
The five-minute rule is only a guide. If things are serious, or Mom says it's time, get to a hospital immediately.

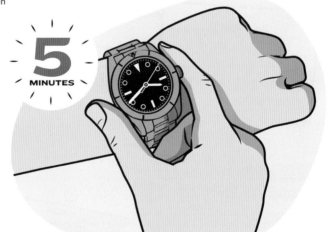

DAD MUST-HAVE: WRISTWATCH

If you've been looking for a reason to purchase a nice dive watch, being an expectant father is as valid as it gets. Part of being Dad involves a) knowing what time it is, all the time, and b) keeping everyone on schedule. This starts with checking the exact moment your baby is born. Be ready.

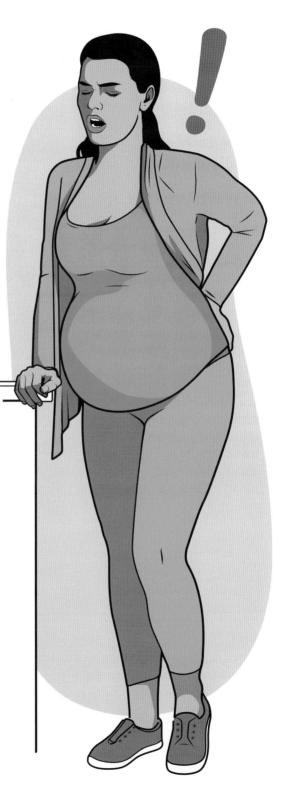

Bloody show

When the mucus plug exits Mom in pieces or at once, labor is usually in her near future.

(4)

Water breaks

The classic sign that the baby's on their way. If the amniotic sac breaks, get to the hospital!

(5)

Backache/cramps

There's more lower back pain than usual and she feels cramps similar to those she experiences when menstruating. Don't ignore this one—call your doctor. It could be caused by "lightening," when the baby descends into the pelvis.

(6)

Diarrhea

Mom's body may release hormones called prostaglandins which may cause frequent (and pungent) trips to the toilet. Her body's trying to get her uterus to begin contractions.

(7)

Feeling fatigued or energized

She's either drained or gets a sudden burst of energy and her nesting impulses are manifesting, well, a lot.

How to Make Dad's Chili

It's a smart idea to master a few things in the kitchen or on the grill. But don't worry—you don't need to reinvent a menu every night, if that's not your thing: You can get the job done with a staple or two that family and friends love. Chili is a perfect example. It's a great dish for you to add your own signature flair and you can set it and walk away while it cooks.

Get a slow cooker and follow this easy recipe for Dad's chili, which you can now pass off as a recipe of your own invention. Adjust the ingredient(s) to your taste and see what works best for your hungry crowd.

'TIS THE SEASON

Typically, chili is well received during the colder months, but if you live in a warm climate, you may want to time your chili with a special event like football kickoff or Christmas Eve. Or you can serve it on rainy days to amp up the cozy (if flatulent) vibes.

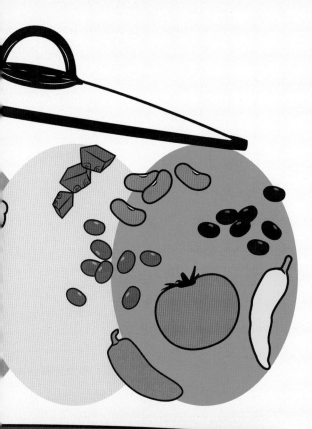

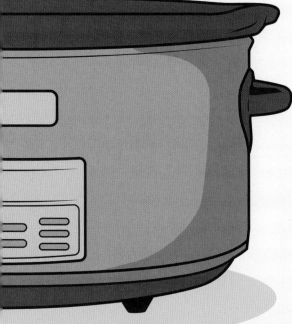

INGREDIENTS

2 lb ground lean beef
1 lb ground turkey
1 chorizo, diced
1 yellow onion, diced
1 can red beans
1 can black beans
1 can kidney beans
2–3 bell peppers (green, red, yellow)
1 jalapeño, diced
1 banana pepper
1 red tomato, diced
8 oz arrabbiata sauce
1 can fire-roasted tomatoes
8 oz BBQ sauce
¼ cup mustard
¼ cup ketchup
Salt, to taste
Pepper, to taste
Chili powder, to taste

DIRECTIONS

Brown the meat a bit alongside the onions, then drain. After that, everything goes into the slow cooker. Cook on low for 6 to 8 hours, stirring occasionally. Serve it in a bowl as is or top it with shredded cheese, sliced avocado or pair it with a grilled cheese sandwich.

Chapter 4

THE BIRTH!

It's like you've been watching nine months of pregame coverage and you've finally arrived at kick-off. You couldn't be any more prepared than you are right now...right? To help ease your anxiety about what to expect inside the delivery room, here's how you and Mom can feel more comfortable.

The Labor and Delivery Room

Your partner has been admitted and assigned to a room and baby's on the way. Congratulations are in order because you're about to officially become a Dad! The delivery room looks a lot like most standard hospital rooms, with a few notable differences. If you didn't already tour the hospital at the beginning of the third trimester, here's your baby birthing room breakdown to mentally prepare yourself for the big day.

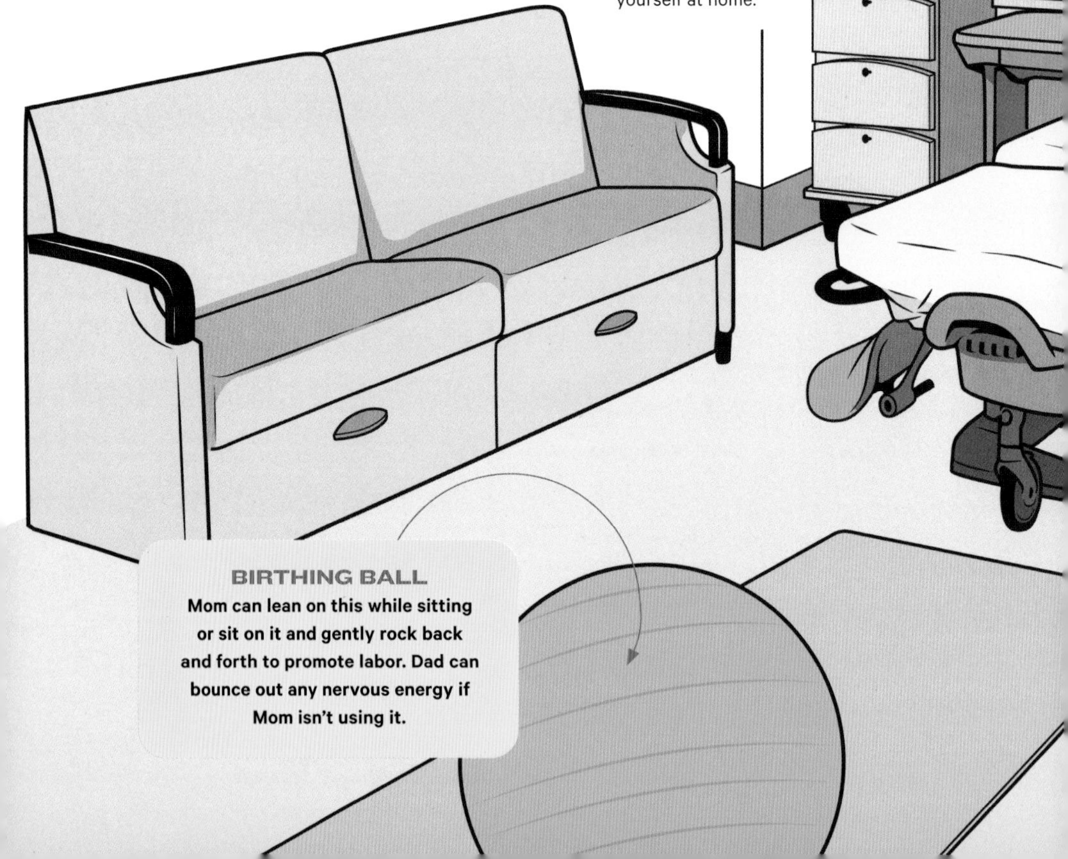

Couch

Sometimes this is just a chair that folds down. Either way, you might be spending the night here, so hope it's comfortable! (If you can sleep, that is.)

Drawers

Space to put your personal items. You may not stay here long, but if you'd like to unpack, make yourself at home.

BIRTHING BALL

Mom can lean on this while sitting or sit on it and gently rock back and forth to promote labor. Dad can bounce out any nervous energy if Mom isn't using it.

Equipment

An incredible amount of medical equipment is tucked away neatly and discreetly in labor and delivery rooms in case of emergencies. DO NOT touch anything!

NURSE'S STATION

When a nurse or doctor enters the room, they typically head straight to the computer to assess the latest readings and diagnostics. The baby is running the show at this point, but lots of data is being collected to help the hospital staff know what's happening at all times.

Bed

These break down in the middle to become birthing beds, complete with stirrups, handles and possibly a birthing bar. Definitely not your average bed.

Fetal monitor

Baby will be getting their own heart rate monitor upon check-in, which will be checked constantly during labor.

Infant warmer

Your baby may or may not end up here. It's a staple of the delivery room with tools to warm the baby up, clear their lungs or just get them clean after arrival.

Stool

Nope, this isn't for you—it's for the doctor or nurse. Make sure it's available for them when they're in the room.

In Case You Have to Wait a Little Longer...

The process of labor may take a few hours, or even a few days. If this is Mom's first time, probably the latter. This means you may have some more waiting to do, but rest assured—the time spent at the hospital is far from boring.

The doctor may have Mom do a number of exercises to promote labor if needed. Some of these may even involve you, so be ready to help out if needed. You might as well break a sweat too for the sake of solidarity. This is also a good time to review your birth plan with all the nurses and doctors on call. Play music, watch TV, but don't be fooled into thinking this is downtime. Active labor is...active! There will be a lot of coming and going, as well as frequent updates from the nurses and doctor. Pay attention and be ready to jump into action.

PASSWORD, PLEASE
After arriving at the hospital, you'll be on your phone quite a bit letting people know all the updates. It's a good idea to connect to the Wi-Fi and save that password so no one misses out due to bad service.

1.
Get the music going
Having music playing at a low level can help set the mood and soothe Mom. Maybe don't lead with the birth playlist, though, as it could be a very long labor. Also remember that songs can have emotional triggers. If Mom's already in a rough state, choose some music that will elevate the room's mood.

2.
Play a game
A traditional board game might be a bit clumsy for the L&D room, but a deck of cards will do just fine. There are plenty of simple card games two people can play, and it might be a good time to brush up on your Go Fish strategy.

3.
Call/text friends and family
Sending out a "before the storm" hospital selfie is a fun way to sound the alarm. Friends and family love to be included, and this may be your last chance before baby arrives to share a message from a simpler, calmer time.

4.
Watch a movie
Depending how fast or slow things are moving, a movie could be a great way to pass a couple hours. Just make sure you know what you're getting into—you wouldn't watch *Final Destination* on a flight, so don't watch *Rosemary's Baby* in the L&D room.

EXERCISES MOM MAY DO TO PROMOTE LABOR

A birthing ball can provide a lot of comfort before and during labor. If Mom is experiencing back pain or discomfort, the ball can provide some relief. But first, ask the nurses and doctor to get a vetted list of what Mom can do.

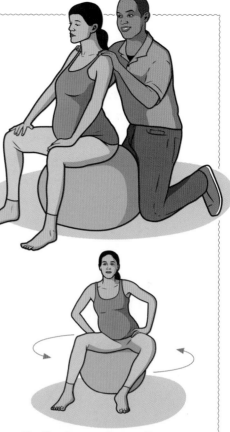

Back support
Mom can sit on the birthing ball as you position yourself behind her to give support. Massage Mom's neck, back or whatever she requests as needed.

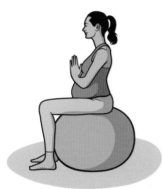

Calm and clear
Mom might want to take a moment to meditate. She can sit up straight, take deep breaths and enjoy the quiet.

She likes to move it move it
As she sits balanced on the ball, Mom can move her hips in a circular motion. This can help get baby ready for labor, too.

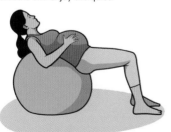

Weight reliever
With her back on the ball, Mom can take a load off by leaning with her knees and hips at a 90-degree angle. Dad can serve as a spotter and help mom back to her feet.

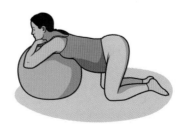

Pressure reliever
Getting on all fours will take pressure off of Mom's lower back and pelvis. She can hug or cradle the ball as needed.

Dilation vs. Effacement

These are two of the buzziest words you'll hear in the time before labor begins. Dilation refers to the size of the opening of the cervix, and effacement is when the cervix softens and thins in preparation for delivery. Doctors monitor both of these metrics to determine when the birthing

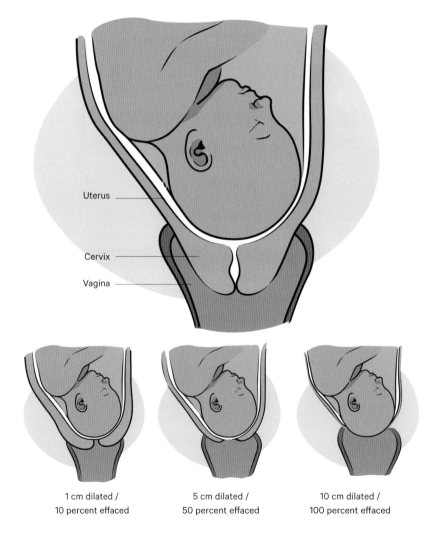

Uterus

Cervix

Vagina

1 cm dilated /
10 percent effaced

5 cm dilated /
50 percent effaced

10 cm dilated /
100 percent effaced

process can begin. Should your medical team decide Mom needs to dilate faster, they may introduce a drug called Pitocin to induce labor and speed things up.

It's crucial that your partner be fully dilated (10 cm) and 100 percent effaced before they start pushing through their contractions, otherwise the baby will not be able to pass through the birth canal and Mom will have to have a Cesarean section (see pg. 106). This is probably a good time to note that Mom has no control over how quickly this happens—it's not something anyone can consciously do, and it's all up to how her body fares during this time. The best thing you can do is keep a cool head and help your partner manage her stress levels.

Regardless of your birth plan, labor for first-time mothers usually takes from 4 to 8 hours, but it can stretch on for more than a day. Thankfully, you're not in this alone—you're surrounded by a team of medical professionals, and you should feel comfortable trusting their cues and advice. If they're not alarmed, you shouldn't be, either.

see pg. 106

DILATION PROGRESS

Dilation can occur rapidly or slowly over many days. But 10 cm is considered fully dilated and ready for baby to pass through. No idea what 10 cm looks like? Here's how a doctor measures:

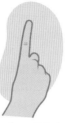
1 cm dilated

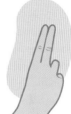
2 cm dilated

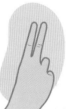
3 cm dilated

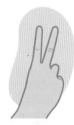
5 cm dilated

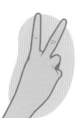
7 cm dilated

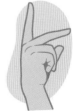
10 cm dilated

CAUTION!
Do not do this yourself. An exam should only be performed by a doctor.

What Is an Epidural?

According to Cleveland Clinic, more than 50 percent of hospital births involve moms who elect to have epidurals. An epidural is a numbing medication injected into Mom's epidural space (the fluid surrounding her spinal cord) via a small catheter to make the process of birthing a baby less painful. This process involves a larger-than-average needle and has some major benefits:

• The medicine is confined to your partner's spine, meaning it won't affect your baby.

• Mom can be awake and mentally present for the delivery.

• Pain management is easily administered and can be felt in minutes.

You'll probably be asked to leave the room, because the environment will need to be kept sterile. While you're out, an anesthesiologist or registered nurse anesthetist will hook Mom up to an IV drip, then sanitize the injection site before administering local anesthesia to

HEADS UP
Dads are typically asked to leave the room, so don't take it personally.

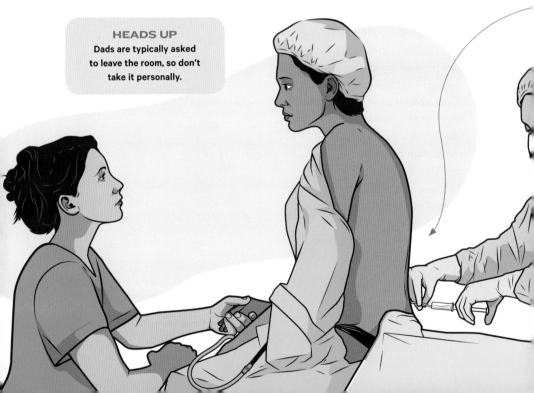

minimize discomfort. Next, with Mom either slouched forward or lying on her side, they'll use the freakishly large (slightly kidding!) needle to insert a thin, flexible tube into Mom's back, a catheter access point for the medicine that will numb Mom from the waist down within 30 minutes. It will remain in her back until shortly after she gives birth, and she can request continuous doses of the numbing agent throughout her labor. Good news: Mom can request an epidural at any time, but earlier on is preferred so that she can feel the relief.

If Mom's having a scheduled Cesarean section (see pg. 106), Mom's epidural will consist of a one-time injection called a spinal block (no catheter needed) to numb her from the breasts down.

After the epidural, the medical staff will supply Mom with a bladder catheter so she can relieve herself during labor.

Side effects can include...
- Feeling itchy all over (don't worry, there's medicine for this)
- Low blood pressure
- Severe headache
- Nausea
- Nerve damage

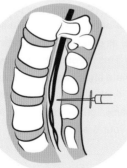

Detail of epidural precision

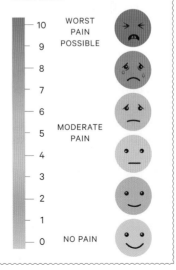

PAIN CHART

If you're curious about how painful labor is and what impact the epidural has, show mom this typical pain chart. Where is she before the epidural, where is she after?

10	WORST PAIN POSSIBLE
9	
8	
7	
6	
5	MODERATE PAIN
4	
3	
2	
1	
0	NO PAIN

What to Do When Mom Is Ready to Push

The doctor will be coming in to take measurements and evaluate both Mom and baby regularly. Based on how everyone is doing, the doctor may make recommendations; but if everything is looking good, a vaginal birth is preferred by everyone.

If labor has progressed to the point where Mom is fully dilated and effaced, it's time for baby to meet you face-to-face. At this point, Mom will want to find a breathing pattern that allows her and baby to relax as much as possible. For some, that may be deep breaths, while others might prefer lighter breathing. After what could be several hours, contractions should become more regular and it will finally be time to push. During a contraction, Mom will push several times. They say to "push like you're pooping" (and she might be doing that, too), so Mom will to bear down like she's having a major bowel movement. If she's able to change positions, that can be helpful. Between contractions, it's a good idea for Mom to rest in order to regain some strength.

So what's Dad doing during all of this? Dad is doing whatever the hell Mom and the doctors tell him to do. Without hesitation, he should be at the ready to provide whatever is needed. This can include helping Mom with breathing exercises, distracting her from the pain or offering a hand, arm or shoulder to clutch during the contractions. It's also a good idea to pay very close attention to the nurses. They do this every day, and if they see Mom responding to you, you may very well become their communication conduit.

Don't shy away from the moment. While you may physically be out of the spotlight, you are there as part of the supporting cast. This is bound to be very intimate and rewarding for your relationship, and seeing Mom in this new light will be forever etched into your brain.

BREATHING WITH MOM

As a show of support, Dad can breathe along with Mom in the same patterns. Do so gently, though—now's not the time to hyperventilate.

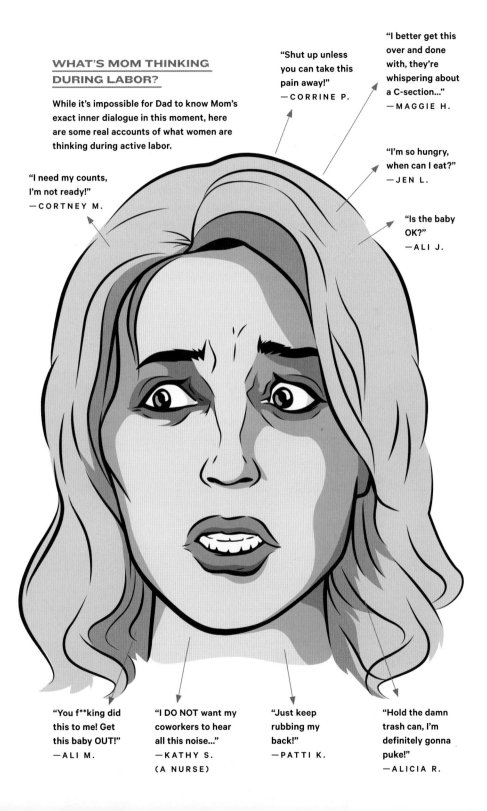

WHAT'S MOM THINKING DURING LABOR?

While it's impossible for Dad to know Mom's exact inner dialogue in this moment, here are some real accounts of what women are thinking during active labor.

"Shut up unless you can take this pain away!"
—CORRINE P.

"I better get this over and done with, they're whispering about a C-section..."
—MAGGIE H.

"I'm so hungry, when can I eat?"
—JEN L.

"Is the baby OK?"
—ALI J.

"I need my counts, I'm not ready!"
—CORTNEY M.

"You f**king did this to me! Get this baby OUT!"
—ALI M.

"I DO NOT want my coworkers to hear all this noise..."
—KATHY S. (A NURSE)

"Just keep rubbing my back!"
—PATTI K.

"Hold the damn trash can, I'm definitely gonna puke!"
—ALICIA R.

Doing It the Old-Fashioned Way

If everyone is healthy and all is going according to plan, you're likely going to have a vaginal birth: exciting!

Now that you've timed Mom's contractions and it's finally time to head to the hospital, Act 1 is over.

From now on the professionals will play the leading role, but your job is far from over. You, however, are the least important person in the room from here on out: get used to the idea. Mom and baby are going to be under extremely close supervision, so the most important thing you can do is help with breathing exercises and assist with

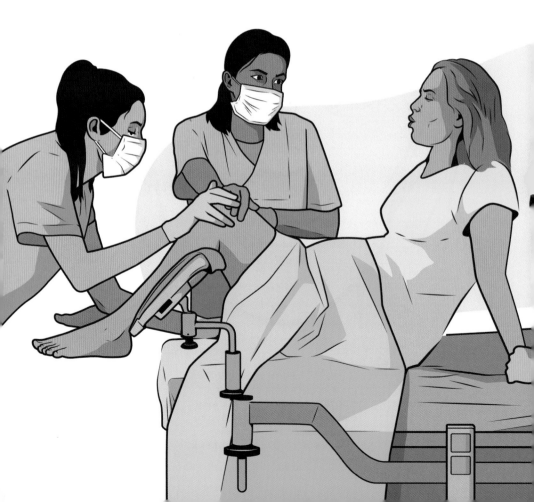

short walks up and down the hall.

Just know that Mom may need to use the bathroom once per hour so her bladder doesn't create a speed bump for baby's head. Then, when contractions are less than a minute apart, it's time to help her push.

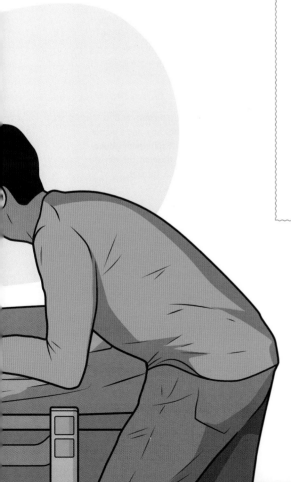

THE HOME STRETCH

Your baby is about to be born, meaning a ton will be happening in a short amount of time. Your job now is to be as close to Mom, baby or both as you can.

Cutting the cord
You might be asked to help cut the umbilical cord. Be prepared for a little blood if you accept.

Clean & clear
Depending on how the delivery goes, baby might go straight to Mom or undergo a quick cleaning and lung clearing beforehand. If you're allowed, you might want to go with baby while the doctors tend to Mom.

Skin-to-skin
After Mom gets her first skin-to-skin contact with baby, it'll be your turn. You'll want to wear a button-down shirt to facilitate this important moment.

AFTERBIRTH
After the baby, the uterus discharges the placenta and fetal membranes. You might see this, you might not. Either way, it still happens and may not be for the light of heart. If you don't like to see blood, stay with the baby and Mom's head.

Cesarean Birth, Explained

Also called a "C-section," this procedure entails Mom delivering the baby through an incision in her abdomen as opposed to vaginally through the birth canal. These can be scheduled ahead of time, but it's not uncommon for a doctor to opt for a C-section on the day of delivery, especially if your partner already had one. Depending on how Mom and baby are doing during labor—namely, if someone's blood pressure is too high or low or if labor stalls or goes on too long—your doctor may choose this procedure over vaginal delivery. This is also what will happen in the event of an emergency, in which case Mom will be whisked into the operating room and everything will move very fast.

Keep in mind: This is major surgery. Your partner may spend two to four days in the hospital, and her recovery at home will require more work on your part in terms of lifting things, helping her take the stairs, etc. The end result? A healthy baby and a badass battle scar.

REASONS FOR AN UNPLANNED OR EMERGENCY C-SECTION

Sometimes a C-section is necessary to ensure Mom and baby stay healthy. Here are some things that may prompt this outcome:

Placenta problems
When it turns out the placenta is partially or completely covering the cervix, **placenta previa** is a potentially life-threatening complication that can cause severe bleeding. Mom will need ample bed rest. **Placental abruption**—aka when the placenta separates from the uterine wall, potentially depriving the baby of vital nutrients and oxygen—will also necessitate a C-section.

Baby in breech
If the baby's sitting feet- or butt-first in the birth canal and a doctor can't manage to turn them around to a head-first position, there's only one way out: through Mom's abdomen.

Umbilical cord prolapse
When the umbilical cord is drooping out of Mom's nether regions, it cuts off the blood flow to the baby, which can be harmful to your little one.

Stalled labor
Whether baby's firmly lodged in place because they're too large to pass through, the cervix isn't fully dilated or Mom's too exhausted to keep pushing, vaginal birth is not an option.

Not for the faint of heart

Be warned, Dad: If a team of doctors is cutting your partner open, you're going to be standing a few feet away from a downright grisly scene. Do not peek past the screen if you're squeamish.

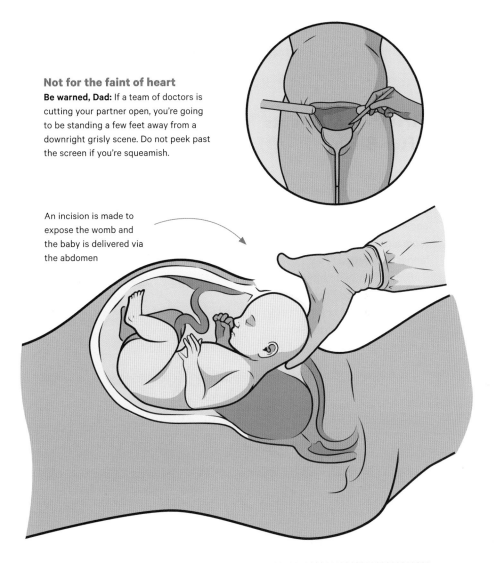

An incision is made to expose the womb and the baby is delivered via the abdomen

TURNING A BABY IN BREECH

If your baby is in breech, the doctor may attempt to maneuver it by performing an external cephalic version (ECV), in which they'll place their hands on Mom's abdomen and attempt to push them into position. But this doesn't always work.

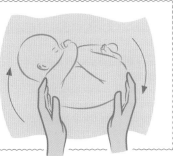

First Few Moments After Birth

Most babies breathe and cry within a few seconds of being born. If it's been a long labor, a pediatrician may be in the birthing room already and help clean baby's lungs if needed.

If your baby is breathing well, they can be placed naked, skin-to-skin, on Mom's chest or belly immediately after birth. Skin-to-skin contact keeps your baby warm, helps steady your baby's breathing and heart rate, and lets Mom and baby bond physically. It's also a trigger for breastfeeding, and baby will be hungry in no time.

Keep in mind, Dad, your kid is coming out of a human body and their skin might be blue

A MESSY ARRIVAL

There's a lot coming out of mom during delivery, but it's all part of the experience of childbirth. If Mom urinates, vomits or poops, don't think twice. These things happen, and there's little she can control.

and mottled. They are likely to be covered in a cheesy white substance called vernix, amniotic fluid and blood. This is normal. Their skin will gain its normal hue as they start to breathe, which is about a minute after birth.

If it's an uncomplicated vaginal birth, the midwife or nurse may dry your baby and clean off some of the bodily fluids with a warm blanket or towel.

If you wish, you can ask to help

EPISIOTOMY

Occasionally a doctor may need to make a cut in the area between the vagina and anus (perineum) during the birth. This is called an episiotomy. The procedure makes the opening of the vagina a bit wider, allowing the baby to arrive more easily.

with the cleaning process, but make sure to defer to the experts.

If your baby was stuck in the vaginal canal or if a vacuum was used, their head may be elongated and alien-like. This is common and the head will return to a normal shape in a few days.

After your baby is born, the umbilical cord will be clamped by a nurse or doctor, and sometime within the first few minutes the cord will be cut to officially separate baby from Mom.

The placenta and afterbirth is disposed of by medical staff, and the doctor will begin working on stitching up mom and making sure any trauma from the birth is treated.

Once Mom and baby are both healthy and healing, you'll notice fewer people in the room, and you'll have time to spend with Mom and baby to count toes, fingers and make the official introductions.

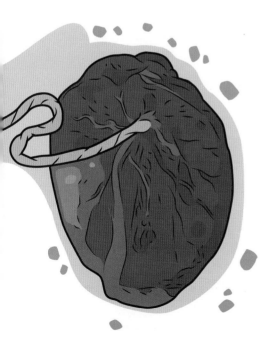

The NICU

During pregnancy, a developing baby is entirely dependent on Mom's body, and the sudden transition to the outside world can be jarring—the light, the sudden temperature change, the noise. It's not uncommon for newborns to need a little extra help learning to breathe amidst all this sensory overload, and that's OK. Don't panic if you hear the doctors mention the NICU in the hectic moments after birth. Over the next few days, your baby will be under close supervision by professionals: It's important for you to be there, but just as important for you to take time for yourself, away from the beeping monitors. If you feel like you need extra support, don't be afraid to ask, especially if you're in for an extended period of time in the NICU. You may also have to field calls to and from your health-care provider regarding specific conditions or any questions you might have.

In all likelihood, your doctors

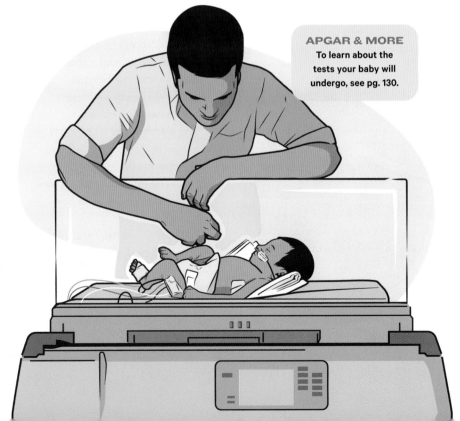

APGAR & MORE
To learn about the tests your baby will undergo, see pg. 130.

ALL THE BEEPING

If you are in the NICU, you will be surrounded by beeping and alerts, which can be a lot to process when it's your baby on the line. Your baby's vital signs monitor is a screen you'll be looking at a lot. Here's a short breakdown of what's what.

(**1**) Heart rate (**2**) Respiration (**3**) Blood pressure (**4**) Oxygen saturation

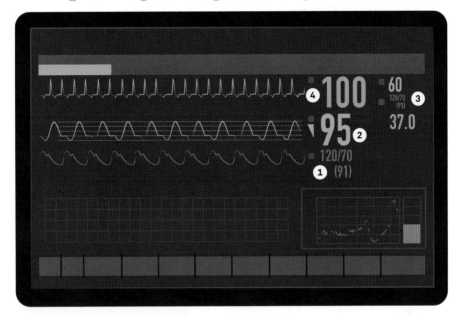

and nurses will have no trouble helping your baby adjust to life beyond this room. So if your birth was premature or otherwise complicated, the NICU is most likely a temporary stop on the way to having a healthy baby at home. In the unlikely event you get bad news, your most important jobs are giving and getting support—in equal measure.

Preparing for Bad News

A lot can go wrong during delivery, and your baby is in a vulnerable place immediately after birth. If you are hit with bad news at any point, embrace loved ones and go where you are needed. If you and your family need counseling or advice about a particular condition, ask your health-care provider for more information.

HAVE SOME TOWELS AROUND
It's a good idea to throw some towels in your car, maybe next to the first aid kit, tire iron and hand sanitizer.

How to Deliver a Baby in the Event of an Emergency

If everything goes according to plan, you won't be delivering your own baby. But if your partner's water has already broken, her contractions are one to two minutes apart, she feels a strong need to push and you or she can already see the baby's head coming (crowning), all while you're still in the car, you're probably not going to make it to the hospital in time. Here's what to do if Mom starts to give birth while you're on the road.

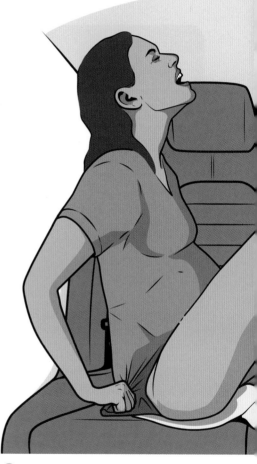

1

Call 911 immediately
The goal is to make sure Mom and baby stay safe throughout delivery. Unless you're a doctor, you are in no way qualified to deliver a baby on your own. Call 911, put the phone on speaker and let them help talk you through the steps one at a time.

2

Turn your hazards on and pull off of the road
This is not the time to be worried about traffic. Turn your hazards on and make sure you safely pull off to the side of the road as soon as possible.

3

Keep Mom comfortable
Depending on how far along her contractions are, you may want to help Mom into the back seat—or let her stay where she is. Focus on helping Mom breathe through the contractions.

4
Hands off

Do not attempt to put your hands anywhere near the birth canal in any way, or you could risk giving Mom or baby an infection.

5
Watch what happens

Now's not the time to be squeamish: Let the dispatcher know what you're seeing, especially if the baby's feet are coming out first, the umbilical cord is wrapped around their neck or Mom's bleeding is excessive, so they can walk you through administering the help your family needs.

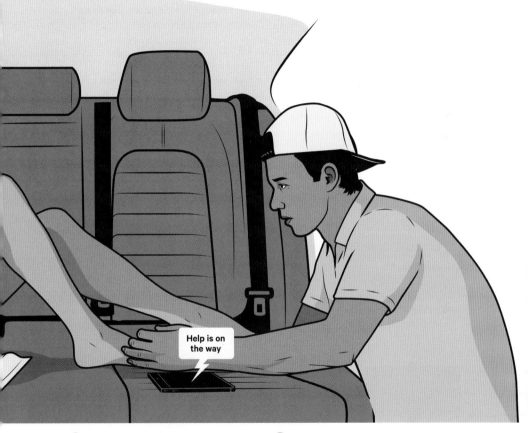

6
No baths just yet

Once the baby is born, do not attempt to wash them off or clean out their ears, eyes, mouth or nose—let the experts handle that later at the hospital. Gently pat them dry with a clean cloth or T-shirt, then lay them on Mom for skin-to-skin contact (under her shirt on her chest is best).

7
Leave the cord alone

There's no need to touch let alone cut the umbilical cord unless medical personnel direct you to do so.

How to Take Better Photos and Videos

One of your implied jobs as Dad is to be ready to record any moment at a moment's notice. Dads of yesteryear used home movie cameras like Super 8s and, later, camcorders to capture family memories on film and VHS, and now it's your turn. Be on the lookout for big firsts, general cuteness or anything else you want to look back on someday, and keep these tips in mind to take photos and videos you'll be proud to rewatch.

1

Wipe the lens
Many an awesome shot has been ruined by an unknown smudge. Take a second before you begin and clean the lens, ya filthy animal.

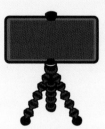

Need a steady shot? Buy a flexible tripod for an extra set of hands.

2

No shadows
If you're outside, put your subject—aka your kiddo—in direct sunlight, facing the sun (but not looking into it, please). If your subject has their back to the sun, they will be backlit and appear very dark in the image, which is a no-go.

3

Front and center
Until you know how to get fancy with framing, stick with the basics by putting your child or Mom or the family pet (or all three!) in the center of the frame. Get as close as possible without invading their personal space and without resorting to zooming in, which makes the picture grainy.

(4)

Beat the clock

It's easy to forget you can all be in the shot (!) if your smartphone has a timer option. Have everyone get into position, set the timer, pray everyone stays where they are and you're golden. If not, try again.

(5)

Action over static

No one's going to begrudge you thousands of photos of your kid sitting or standing there looking adorable. But capturing the moment your child decides to drape themselves in their spaghetti or play with the family pet makes for a dynamic subject that comes with a story.

INTERVIEW WITH A TOT

Once they build up enough vocabulary (or maybe before), ask your child basic questions—"How old are you?" "What's your favorite toy?" "Will the Red Sox win this year?"—and record their responses.

Don't forget to save your memories on the cloud so you don't max out space on your phone.

HORIZONTAL WHEN RECORDING

Dad, PLEASE do not be that person who holds their phone vertically when recording video. Landscape (aka horizontal) orientation will present better online as well as on your television if you ever watch it outside of your phone. This is the simplest way to embrace your inner Spielberg.

Chapter 5

THE FIRST 48 HOURS

(OF THE REST OF YOUR LIFE)

The excitement of delivery can prove overwhelming. But once the room calms down, it's time to meet your baby and make some introductions. You'll most likely be in the hospital for a couple of days, during which time you'll take a crash course on parenting as well as wander the halls with zombie-level exhaustion. Thankfully, a helpful team of doctors and nurses will be at your beck and call.

Officially a Dad

Congratulations! You're the world's newest dad, ready to put months of research and training to good use. As the excitement of the delivery and meet-and-greet winds down, your family will be moved to a postpartum room. If possible, request this before the delivery because there are a limited number of private rooms and they get booked up.

Once you're settled in, it's time to get the whole family together for introductions and some good old-fashioned cuddling. Baby wants to do two things: eat and sleep (sometimes simultaneously). Mom may try breastfeeding. You, unfortunately, can't be much help here. Instead, spend all your time learning baby care basics by listening to the nurses and doctors.

It's a truly wonderful time, and you may have a lot of questions. Good news is, you're not alone. Many men before you have had the same prevailing thoughts in the moments after the baby is born.

Note: Now that you've finished this paragraph, you are no longer the world's newest dad.

"Are these his permanent features or will he change once he's out of the infant stage?"
—ANDY B.

What can I do to help?

My phone's been blowing up—when is it OK to let people know baby has arrived?

"How long before he's housebroken?"
—MARTY C.

Is the baby getting enough to eat? How do we know?

"Is this how my parents felt? This instant, boundless love for this tiny human?"
—JOE B.

Am I doing a good job?

I just saw some crazy shit in that delivery room. How's Mom doing? When will she be completely healed?

DAD HACK
If you live close enough to the hospital, and Mom approves (or if you have someone to help cover during your absence, like Grandma), slip out for a power nap at home. You'll get more quality rest in order to be your best self. Just hustle back to the hospital ASAP!

YOU MIGHT HAVE SOME QUESTIONS...

"The nurses can come home with us, right?"
—GLEN K.

Why is the baby's head all long and weird looking?

I'm exhausted, when can I sleep?

Is my baby healthy?

"When will we feel normal, not nervous, as parents?"
—DREW R.

Uhmmmmm uh, uhm...now what?

A Revolving Door of Assistance

Even if you have little to no experience with babies, you're about to get a lot of practice in a very safe environment where professionals are ready to jump in at a moment's notice to keep you from holding your baby by its darling cheeks. Be ready to take notes and get as many pointers as you can.

Ask lots of questions

Pay close attention to the nurses and ask them anything and everything. The information you'll be getting from the hospital staff during this part of your stay is invaluable. These nurses are experts and they will gladly share their knowledge. Not sure how to put on the diaper? Ask. Don't know where to put the diaper cream? Speak up. Unsure what colostrum is? Ask the lactation consultant for a quick breakdown. Not sure why you need a lactation consultant? Ask your partner. Take advantage of the professional help that surrounds you before you head home and rely on Google to fill in the rest.

There will be paperwork

In addition to hospital billing paperwork, there's a birth certificate, social security registration and more documents you'll be required to complete before leaving the hospital. No need to bring your own pen, but be ready to captain this responsibility. Note: If your baby doesn't have a name at this stage, take a breath and talk it through. You don't want to put "TBD" on any federal forms.

Remember that empty duffel bag

The hospital will provide diapers (for baby and Mom), wipes and miscellaneous baby gear. Whatever is not used can be taken with you when you leave, so stock up.

Bring thank-you cards

A card is a heartfelt touch the whole team will appreciate.

Share the excitement

Family and friends are on pins and needles waiting to hear the good news, so if you have time, make sure to update them.

TAKE THE LEAD

Ask one of your nurses what you can acquire from elsewhere in the hospital on your own (e.g., water, extra pillows, fruit cups, the TV remote) so you don't have to bug them any time you, baby or Mom has requests.

BABY CUES

Your baby will communicate what they want by smacking their lips, crying, squirming, etc., all of which are indications they want something or feel uncomfortable in some way. You will learn to read these cues like a pitcher reads catcher signs.

COLOSTRUM

This pre-breast milk concentrate (aka liquid gold) comes from Mom's breasts. It's packed with proteins to facilitate baby's development and antibodies to build their immune system.

LACTATION CONSULTANT

The breastfeeding expert who will come around and make sure your baby can latch onto Mom's breast before you leave the hospital.

CIRCUMCISION

Definitely have this discussion with your partner BEFORE she goes into labor, and don't assume the staff will automatically chop off the foreskin—let your physician/team know.

SKIN-TO-SKIN CONTACT

Mom placing baby on her chest (or yours!) will help calm them as well as regulate their body temperature and blood sugar levels. An easy and adorable way to boost oxytocin levels.

NIPPLE SHIELD

As the lactation consultant will explain, despite sounding like an accessory in some avant-garde Captain America fanfic, this is a silicone tool that may help your little one latch on with ease.

JAUNDICE

This is the reason your baby looks like a knock-off Minion. About 60 percent of babies will look more yellow than they should at birth. This condition is usually harmless and goes away on its own; if not, blue light therapy at the hospital does the trick.

How to Hold, Feed and Burp a Baby

TRY NOT TO OVERFEED
A newborn baby's stomach is about the size of a big marble. That's not a lot of volume, so be careful not to overfeed them or it's coming back up.

If Mom is breastfeeding exclusively, you will have to wait to deliver the goods by bottle, but don't worry, that day will come. In the meantime, you'll still need to get used to holding your baby, so be sure to ALWAYS SUPPORT THE HEAD and know you're holding priceless merchandise. Doing anything with a newborn can feel awkward if you've never interacted with a baby before, so watch a nurse first to get the general idea, then ask for supervision the first time you try it (preferably while sitting in a chair). Doing is the best way to learn, so here are the basics.

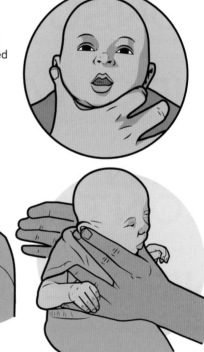

Over-the-shoulder
A classic, cuddly way to get the extra air out: Hold them facing you, lay their head on your shoulder and gently pat their back until they burp.

Chin cradle
Sit the baby on your knee, cradle the chin with one hand and gently pat baby's back until they burp.

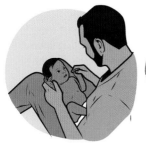

Lap hold

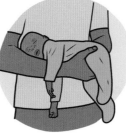

Belly hold

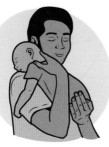

Shoulder hold

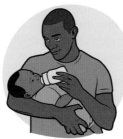

Football hold

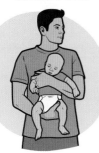

Chair hold

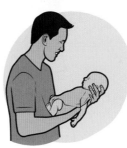

Face-to-face hold

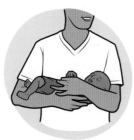

Cradle hold

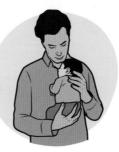

Snuggle hold

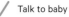

DO

✓ Sanitize hands before holding baby

✓ Grab a towel and be ready for spit-up

✓ Ask for help if needed

✓ Always support the neck

✓ Be very gentle

✓ Talk to baby

✓ Count baby's fingers and toes

DON'T

✗ Bounce or shake baby

✗ Make sudden or quick movements when holding baby

✗ Block or cover baby's mouth and nose with a blanket or swaddle

✗ Be intimidated

✗ Check the day's scores on your phone

How to Change a Diaper

BEWARE THE PEE
A baby can pee or poop without much warning. Place a washcloth over your baby's privates or accept the consequences.

Never changed a diaper before? No problem. You'll soon be doing it in your sleep (almost literally). Part of being a Dad is knowing how to change your baby and keep them clean, so if it's your first rodeo, here's a good visual guide to get you started.

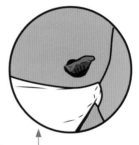

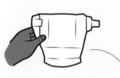

Place fresh diaper under your baby

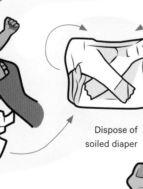

The umbilical cord can take up to three weeks to heal, dry up and fall off. Try your best not to aggravate it, as it may lead to some bleeding. Keep it clean, change diapers frequently, don't poke it and stick to sponge baths until it's gone.

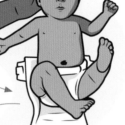

Dispose of soiled diaper

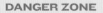

DANGER ZONE

You may have to repeat this step if baby decides to double down on evacuating while being changed, which is common.

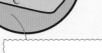

BLOWOUTS

Due to velocity, volume or a precise combination of the two, you will experience occasions where the diaper, despite claims on the packaging, cannot contain your baby's butt stuff. Accept the fact that you may need to give your pride and joy a bath.

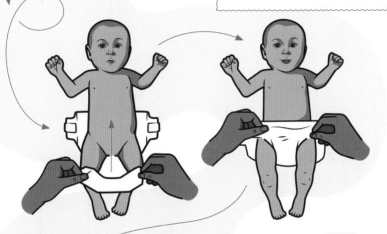

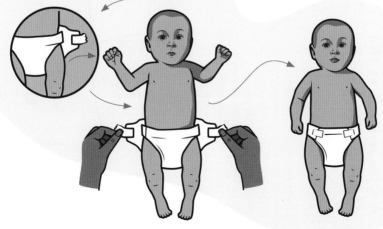

A Closer Look at the Almighty Diaper

Changing your baby will get bothersome, but make no mistake: the diaper is your best friend in the world now. Something that's so important to your life merits a few minutes dedicated to a deeper understanding of its sorcery.

(1) **The waistband**
Made of elastic so baby can move around comfortably.

(2) **The last line of defense**
A thin plastic film protects the absorptive layers from the outside world.

(3) **The fastener**
Usually made of a Velcro-type closure. Make sure it's not touching baby's skin directly.

NOT IN THE POOL
If you take your tot swimming (not recommended under 6 months old) be sure to use a diaper designed for swimming. Putting your baby in a pool with a normal diaper will end poorly.

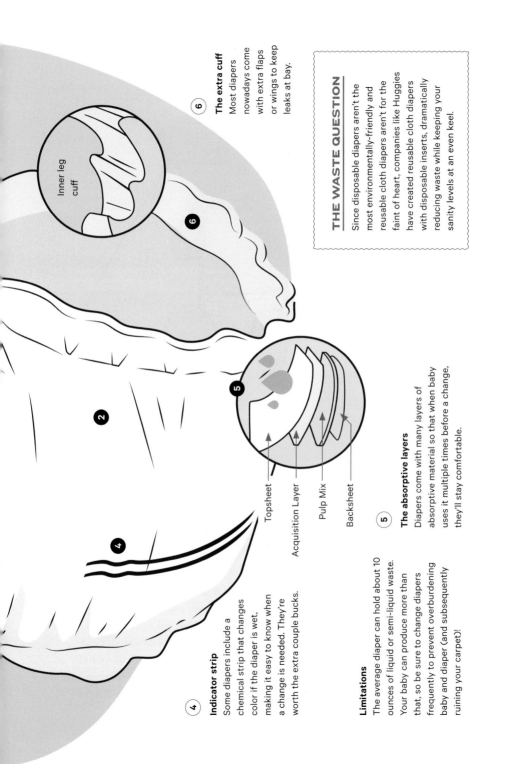

6 The extra cuff

Most diapers nowadays come with extra flaps or wings to keep leaks at bay.

Inner leg cuff

Topsheet
Acquisition Layer
Pulp Mix
Backsheet

4 Indicator strip

Some diapers include a chemical strip that changes color if the diaper is wet, making it easy to know when a change is needed. They're worth the extra couple bucks.

Limitations

The average diaper can hold about 10 ounces of liquid or semi-liquid waste. Your baby can produce more than that, so be sure to change diapers frequently to prevent overburdening baby and diaper (and subsequently ruining your carpet)!

5 The absorptive layers

Diapers come with many layers of absorptive material so that when baby uses it multiple times before a change, they'll stay comfortable.

THE WASTE QUESTION

Since disposable diapers aren't the most environmentally-friendly and reusable cloth diapers aren't for the faint of heart, companies like Huggies have created reusable cloth diapers with disposable inserts, dramatically reducing waste while keeping your sanity levels at an even keel.

How to Swaddle a Baby Like a Pro

For a brief period of time, you can and probably should swaddle your baby. Swaddling helps baby curb their natural startle reflex when resting and prevents their talon-like fingernails from scratching their face. A proper swaddle can also relieve anxiety as it simulates the enclosed comfort of the womb, which baby might miss early on.

Like all baby care, swaddling takes a bit of practice to master. For starters, you'll want to choose a material that has some texture to it—silky fabrics can be difficult for a first-timer, so hold off on baby living their best luxe life for now and start with the hospital-issued cotton fabrics.

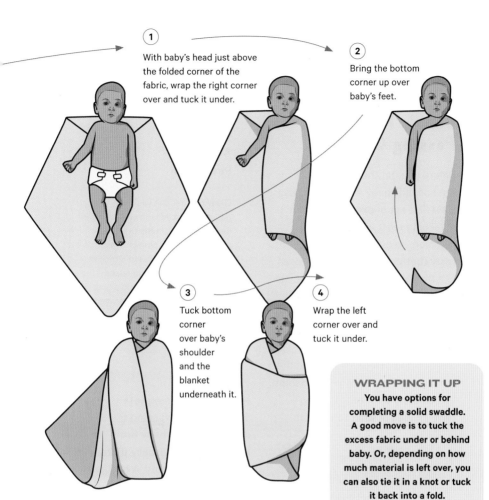

1 With baby's head just above the folded corner of the fabric, wrap the right corner over and tuck it under.

2 Bring the bottom corner up over baby's feet.

3 Tuck bottom corner over baby's shoulder and the blanket underneath it.

4 Wrap the left corner over and tuck it under.

WRAPPING IT UP

You have options for completing a solid swaddle. A good move is to tuck the excess fabric under or behind baby. Or, depending on how much material is left over, you can also tie it in a knot or tuck it back into a fold.

THE CHEAT SHEET

If the old-fashioned way seems too daunting at the moment, you can make things easier by buying a swaddle sack with Velcro or snaps. Follow these steps if you go that route.

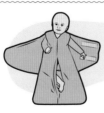
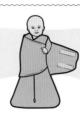
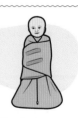

Step 1 Dress baby in regular sleepwear and close the zipper.

Step 2 Fold left swaddle wing over baby's right arm and torso, tucking under baby's left arm.

Step 3 Affix the other wing so the wrap is snug below the chin and aligned with baby's shoulders.

Baby's First Passing Grades

Before you get the all clear to leave the hospital, baby will have to pass their first set of exams. Newborn screening tests are completely common, so don't worry or get testy (better get used to Dad jokes like that: you're about to appreciate them much more). Feel free to ask the medical staff questions if you're not sure what's going on: You'll be seeing a lot of new stuff and it's OK to be curious. Here are a few of the most common tests given to babies immediately after birth, so you'll have an idea of what to expect.

ADVOCATE FOR YOURSELF AND YOUR BABY
Unsure what the hell is going on? Ask questions. Talk to your doctor and make sure you have a full understanding of when your baby is tested and what to expect.

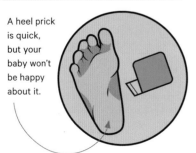

A heel prick is quick, but your baby won't be happy about it.

THE APGAR TEST

Appearance
Pulse
Grimace
Activity
Respiration

Likely the first test your baby will get after birth, APGAR stands for Appearance, Pulse, Grimace, Activity (and) Respiration. It's an observational test that determines your baby's basic life functions are working as they should: things like reflexes, heartbeat, movement and breathing.

Newborn screening test
The newborn screening test is done when your baby turns 24 hours old and is usually performed by the nurse on duty. A heel prick will produce five small blood samples for testing. It can be jarring to see your baby's first blood test, but it's all for the greater good—this test allows the medical staff to make sure baby's body is functioning normally and will check for metabolic diseases, genetic disorders and thyroid problems, among other things. You may also be asked if you'd like to donate any of your baby's sample for future research. This is, of course, entirely up to you.

Hearing test
Sometime in the first day or so after your baby's birth, the medical staff will administer a hearing test. It's not uncommon for residue left over from the birthing process to interfere with the test at first, so don't panic if progress is a bit slower on this test than others.

The bilirubin test
This test only takes a few seconds—it checks for jaundice and will detect if your baby's level of bilirubin is getting too high. Nowadays, this doesn't even involve drawing blood most of the time: a light sensor is used instead.

Near-continuous weighings
Don't be alarmed if your baby gets weighed a lot during the first day or two: The medical staff is not conducting weigh-ins for their underground baby boxing league. They're just gauging whether or not baby is getting enough nutrients based on weight loss.

Getting Baby in the Car Seat

Before you're allowed to leave the hospital, both Mom and baby will need to be in a condition that satisfies the doctor's requirements for discharge (sorry, missing your own bed does not count). Dad will be busy packing up everyone's belongings and readying the car for the trip home, a role that should become very familiar over the next few months and years. Most hospitals require a new baby car seat be purchased for baby's trip home, and both parents will need to know how to get their baby into the seat and securely strapped in before your happy family can leave. Don't mind if baby fusses a bit— they, like you, have had a long few days and still have a lot to learn.

Important reminder:
Make sure you and Mom have your cellphones, keys, ID cards, wallets and any other critical personal items you might have squirreled away during the birthing frenzy before you hop in the car.

> **DETACHABLE BASE**
> **Many car seats have a detachable base. Read the installation instructions carefully and make sure the base and seat are secure before you hit the road.**

BUCKLE UP

It's awkward until it's not, so try to embrace your new routine with dad-ly gusto. Depending on your car seat you could have more or fewer steps than the ones outlined below. Always read all instructions for setting up your rear-facing car seat.

(1) Remove the shoulder strap covers.

(2) Loosen the straps by pulling them toward you and pressing the release button.

(3) Gently place the baby in the car seat and make sure their bottom is touching the inner base of the car seat. You might gently, slowly wiggle them into place to achieve this.

(4) Make sure their chin is up. Avoid the chin-to-chest position, which will make it harder for baby to breathe. Gently turning your newborn's head to one side is recommended.

(5) Fasten clips and buckles as directed for their arms and legs. This may take a few rounds of checking, so take your time and be patient.

(6) Tighten the straps until your baby is snug and secure (big gaps—aka more than two fingers' worth of space between your baby's body and the straps— are no good).

(7) Make sure the chest clip is across their chest, NOT their stomach, otherwise this could damage their internal organs. And they need those.

Cover and swaddle your baby in a blanket from the chest down and neatly tuck them in for comfort and warmth. If they're still fussing, gently tap their chest and speak calmly to them to get them quiet (maybe).

Close (but don't slam!) the door. Wave at your progeny. Marvel at your own magnificence.

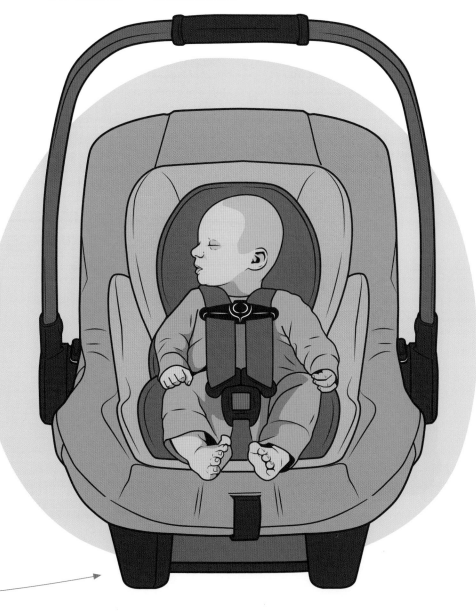

On Your Own

You came here as a couple and are leaving as a party of three (unless you used a surrogate). The car ride from the hospital to your home is surreal to say the least. You've picked up some precious cargo during your stay, and in addition to driving slower/more carefully than you normally would, you'll want to keep your eyes on the road rather than on your cute little bundle of joy.

It's been an intense few days, and the 24/7 support of the hospital staff was comforting to say the least. No longer having the in-

If anyone buys you an oversized bear, they might mean well but they are NOT your friend. Also, don't block the rearview mirror.

Mom may choose to ride in the back seat with baby, which means you've got a visual on your kid at all times. Less work for you!

Baby's carseat should face backwards for the first 2–4 years.

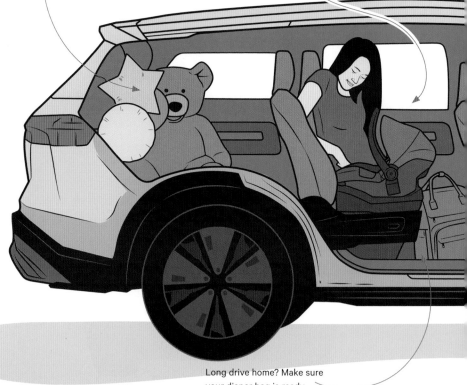

Long drive home? Make sure your diaper bag is ready.

person team of experts may make you feel a bit jumpy, but know that everyone feels this way at first and it won't last forever. You, like your child, will continue to grow and learn and, yes, fail miserably from time to time. Handle them, and yourself, with care. That starts with looking both ways before leaving the hospital parking lot.

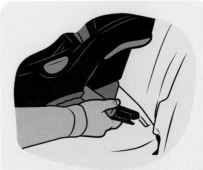

LATCH VS. SEATBELT

There are two ways to secure a baby car seat in your vehicle. The easiest way is to latch the base onto the built-in hooks in the car. If your car doesn't have the built-ins, use the seatbelt to secure the car seat in place.

You might be feeling nervous, tired, anxious and possibly even nauseous on the ride home. That's OK: It will pass.

Your personal bags and free hospital swag are the first things you should have packed in the car.

Make sure the car is in good working order (enough gas, no check engine light on, all four tires, full tank of blinker fluid,* etc.) before you leave the hospital.

*This is one prime Dad Joke for the road.

How to Ride a Motorcycle

Part of being a dad is simply looking cool (or, as often, thinking you look cool). If you're not the jorts and white New Balance type, perhaps you'd prefer to turn heads by zooming by on a motorcycle. But before you actually hit the road on your hog, you have to know exactly what you're doing.

(1)

Gear up

Let's face it: half the reason you want to ride this thing is so you can justify dressing like this. Get yourself a leather jacket (snug in the torso but with good arm mobility), boots (non-slip soles, steel toe), gloves (good finger mobility, wrist straps) and most importantly, a professionally-fitted helmet.

(2)

Climb aboard

While standing on the left side of the bike with your hand on the left handlebar, swing your right leg over the seat. Plant both feet on the ground—they should comfortably reach as they would on a regular bike.

3

Control yourself
You may think you know the controls on a motorcycle just from observing the ones parked at your local dive, but it's imperative to familiarize yourself with these once you're actually sitting on a bike. There's no shame practicing in the parking lot. Well, maybe a little shame.

4

Coming in clutch
Understanding the clutch is crucial. Pulling the clutch releases the motorcycle's engine from the transmission—in other words, it allows you to shift gears by putting the bike in neutral. You'll need to practice the pull (smooth and steady, not an abrupt or forceful squeeze) so you don't stall the bike.

5

Gentlemen, start your engines
To start the bike, insert the key into the ignition. Pull the clutch and flip the red kill switch (usually found on the right handlebar) to the on position. Now turn the key in the ignition, then adjust the clutch until the bike is in neutral (indicated by the "N" on the gauge lighting up). Push the start button—typically found under the kill switch and marked with a circular arrow and lightning bolt—and let the bike warm up for about 45 seconds after the engine turns over. Keeping your feet flat on the ground, pull the clutch in. Use your heels to roll back, then repeat this several times to get used to the clutch.

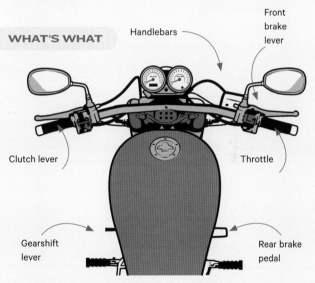

WHAT'S WHAT

Handlebars

Front brake lever

Clutch lever

Throttle

Gearshift lever

Rear brake pedal

SEEK EXPERTISE

Regardless of whether or not your state requires you to get a license, taking a motorcycle training and safety course is crucial. As appealing as motorcycles are, you have to remember how dangerous they can be, too. Don't go for a spin until you've had plenty of practice under the guidance of an expert.

Chapter 6

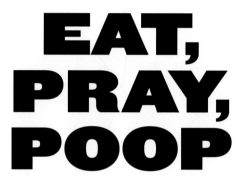

EAT, PRAY, POOP

Just when you think you've got things down, you're back at home and on your own. Brace yourselves to reach out for help and prepare for all of your lives to revolve around sleeping, eating and pooping.

The Poo-Petual Cycle

The first days after you arrive home might be a sleep-deprived blur, but chin up: Your baby will soon fall into a routine of eating, pooping and sleeping—sometimes all at once! In the meantime, harness the power of habit by practicing your diaper-changing and swaddling skills. Here's what an average day might look like for your new little family.

6:00 A.M.
Baby doesn't know what morning or night is (and you might be muddled, too), so let's say your day begins bright and early.

6:30 A.M.
After their first feeding of the day, your baby burps, eats a little more and dozes back off to sleep. Have a cup of coffee.

6:45 A.M.
Baby wakes up because they pooped! A quick diaper change and back to sleep (them, not you).

9:45 A.M.
More eating! Have a protein power snack.

10:00 A.M.
More pooping! Are you picking up on how quickly baby bowel movements occur, yet?

10:30 A.M.
Looks like your little one's hungrier than you thought. More eating!

10:45 A.M.–2:30 P.M.
Hopefully you'll get some good long stretches where your baby is sound asleep. Take advantage of this by having lunch, running errands, cleaning or catching some z's. You earned it.

2:35 P.M.
You're gonna need a bigger diaper—cue poopageddon. Looks like it's bath time!

3:35 P.M.
The extended nap means your baby chows down, burps and eats some more (careful not to overfeed, though).

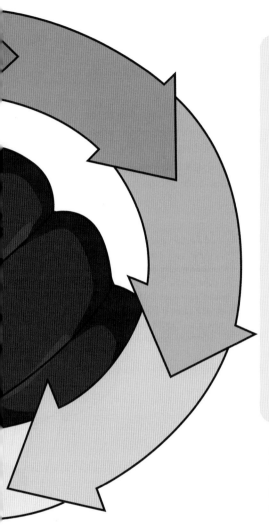

HOW DO YOU KNOW YOUR BABY HAS POOPED?

After a while, you just know. Sometimes, it's a mystery. Sometimes, it's gas. But all your senses can help you determine if baby is in need of a diaper change. Except taste...don't do that.

You sense the telltale smell of fresh poo

You see baby's scrunchy workin' face, or poop

You hear baby grunting (or a squishy diaper)

You feel the warmth and heft of a full load

9:30 P.M.–1:30 A.M.
The hope is for baby to sleep for several hours now. Don't count on it. Have a few bottles prepped and be on the lookout for another diaper change.

2:00 A.M.
Someone is awake (no, not you) and they're HANGRY. "Whose turn is it to feed?" you wonder out loud. Trick question: It's always YOURS.

3:45 A.M.
Guess whose bowel movement startled them awake! Hopefully baby's!

5:00 A.M.
Don't you wake up in an hour?
Doesn't matter—the cycle continues!

6:35 P.M.
Dinnertime! Make sure you and Mom are staying hydrated.

8:35 P.M.
Baby's dozed off. Perfect time to hit the couch and sleep through your favorite show.

9:00 P.M.
Today wasn't so bad, you think. What's that spot on your shirt? *Wait...is that poop from earlier?* Change their diaper, then change your top.

Family Helpers and Friends

When it comes to help, take every bit you can. Your siblings, parents or in-laws may drive you crazy, but focus on what they're capable of doing when you're running on empty. Cooking dinner, running errands—these things are usually far more helpful than having someone hold the baby. People are often eager to jump in but don't want to overstep, so don't be afraid to ask someone to do something outright: "We really need some fruits and veggies to have on hand for snacks—mind running to the store? Here's a list." Alternatively, don't feel bad if you want them to watch the baby like a hawk for an hour while you go run errands

> **BE AT THE READY**
> Dad can be extra helpful if he acts as the at-your-service concierge for Mom and guests. Make sure everyone is comfortable, has a place to sit, and knows where the bathroom is located, as well as what the new rules of the house are (which you should take a minute to establish with Mom).

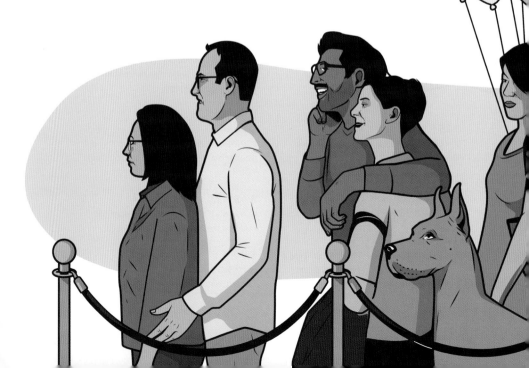

if that little escape helps you feel human again. Be upfront about what you need and trust everyone to do the rest. Here are some tasks to get the welcome crew started.

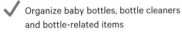 Organize baby bottles, bottle cleaners and bottle-related items

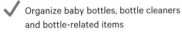 Wash baby clothes (or your clothes, if you're close); cut tags off items as needed

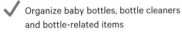 Set up baby monitor, assemble baby items as needed

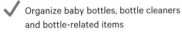 Video chat with other family members who would like to virtually meet the baby

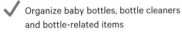 Buy food (and, if desired, some booze) and/or meal prep

INTRODUCING YOUR PET

Here's how to have your fur baby greet your actual offspring.

The old baby blanket trick
Offer your pet a sniff of your baby's blanket to get them acquainted via scent. If it's not love at first whiff, that's OK. Building relationships takes time.

The meet-cute
Allow your pet to spend a minute or two with Mom first, then with the baby. This is best done outdoors, with a leash and/or a bit of distance, to keep everyone safe.

Pay attention to cues
Is your furry friend's body relaxed and friendly or alert and tense? If it's the former, give LOTS of pats for reinforcement. If it's the latter, don't force it—try again later.

No one-on-one time
No matter how cute either is, never leave your baby and pet unattended.

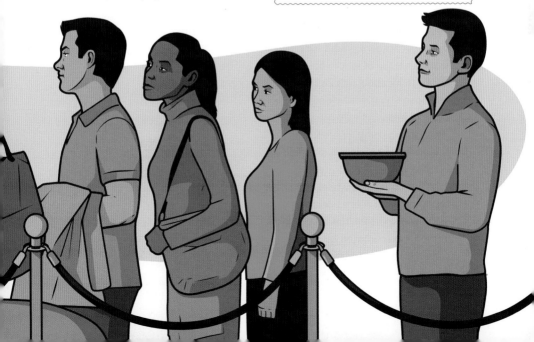

Mental Health Reality Check

You're finally home from the hospital, and acclimating to the schedule dictated by your new housemate's needs is a huge deal. Mom's journey into parenthood is considerably more arduous than yours. In the next few weeks and months, your partner's hormones will settle down from their elevated pregnancy levels and her organs will shift back into their pre-baby positions. In other words: No, the toll of pregnancy did NOT end when she squeezed what felt like a 9-pound watermelon out of her body. If Mom had a C-section, she can't simply bend over and scoop up the baby when they're crying or hungry—Mom needs to recover from major surgery. And it isn't just the physical toll of labor you both need to think about. It's important to be open about your mental health as well.

Even if becoming a parent was something you've always dreamed of, it's OK to feel like your emotions are all over the place while adapting to your role as caregiver. With new responsibilities come new stressors (exacerbated by sleep deprivation and hormone levels), and if you or Mom feel like you're struggling, say something. Check in with your partner, talk about how you're handling the transition and keep an eye out for signs of postpartum depression (PPD), which can linger for weeks and months after delivery. According to Cleveland Clinic, about one in seven new parents will experience PPD, dads included. If you or Mom are exhibiting any of the signs on the right, don't assume things will resolve themselves—contact your doctor right away.

> **"For the first six months of my son's life, I was living in a daze of sleep deprivation, crippling anxiety and inadequacy."**
> —MICHELLE B.

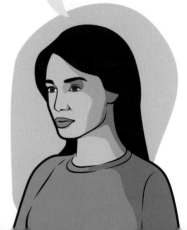

FEELING GUILTY

Or profound feelings of desperation, dread, hopelessness, panic or worthlessness. This is different for everyone, but one thing's for sure: No one deserves to feel it.

ANXIETY

Pacing, excessive worrying, and feeling on edge, irritable, overwhelmed or like you're stuck in fight-or-flight mode are all signs that something's not right. It might even be a case of **postpartum anxiety**, which your doctor can diagnose.

LOSS OF APPETITE

A solid indication of a major chemical shift in one's hormones. If it lasts longer than two weeks, it's a problem.

FREQUENT CRYING

Imagine mood swings on steroids. This might also look like crying for no reason. Not pleasant for anyone and the bluest red flag in the bunch.

TRAUMATIC CHILDBIRTH

If delivering the baby was a rough (read: life-threatening or complication-laden) experience, Mom is at greater risk of developing PPD.

CONCERNING THOUGHTS

If you or Mom are gripped by thoughts of suddenly not wanting your baby or harming yourself or your baby, seek immediate medical help.

Breast Pumps

Ah, the sound of the breast pump. It's a noise you won't soon forget. If you're fortunate enough to have a hands-free pump, Mom can seamlessly incorporate milk expressing into her daily multitasking routine (or take a well-deserved opportunity to just sit and let the machine do its thing). During those first few weeks post-delivery, the breast pump will feel like a major part of your support crew, especially while Mom gets to work turning the freezer into a Fort Knox full of liquid gold.

To keep things running smoothly, make sure to organize those rows of gleaming bottles in an orderly

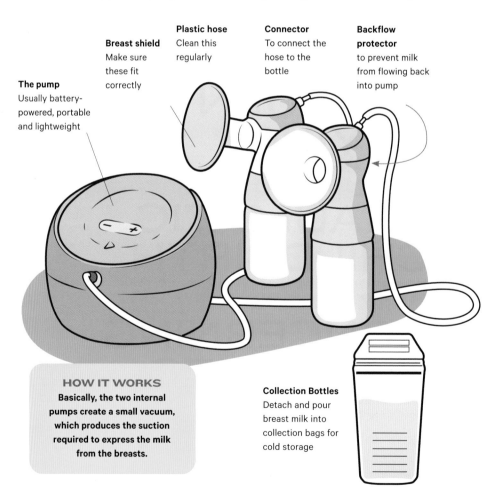

Plastic hose
Clean this regularly

Breast shield
Make sure these fit correctly

Connector
To connect the hose to the bottle

Backflow protector
to prevent milk from flowing back into pump

The pump
Usually battery-powered, portable and lightweight

HOW IT WORKS
Basically, the two internal pumps create a small vacuum, which produces the suction required to express the milk from the breasts.

Collection Bottles
Detach and pour breast milk into collection bags for cold storage

fashion, rotating the freshest milk to the back, always grabbing the older milk first. Whenever pump issues happen, you and your partner should know how to troubleshoot the device, so read the instructions carefully. In general, make sure the connections are tight and there are no cracks in the tubing or shields. If it's still

ODDLY ENOUGH…
Bodybuilders buy breast milk. It's packed full of muscle-building nutrients and proteins, and serious contenders will pay up for Mom's natural product by the ounce.

not working, try disassembling the valves and membranes, cleaning all the parts, then reassembling. If that doesn't work, buy another pump immediately. No dallying—once Mom begins producing milk, she'll need to pump!

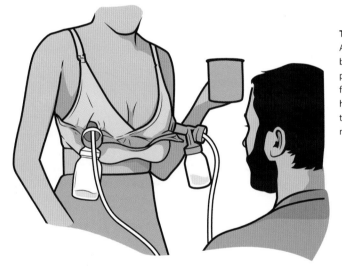

The big sexy
A pumping bra can make pumping a hands-free, minimal hassle experience that you can never unsee.

MASTITIS AND A BLOCKED MILK DUCT

Clogged milk ducts are no one's idea of a good time, but they happen. These small, tender lumps in Mom's breast can usually be treated with a warm, moist compress and/or an over-the-counter pain reliever, and voilà, back to normal.

But if that doesn't work, an untreated blocked milk duct will typically lead to breast inflammation, aka mastitis. This can be very painful and can even cause Mom to experience flu-like symptoms. If she's still feeling the pain within 12–24 hours of first noticing it, or if she starts to feel worse, it's time to call a doctor. She may need to take a course of antibiotics.

Bath Time!

Until baby's umbilical cord falls off (10–14 days after birth), it's a good idea to just give the kid a sponge bath. Since babies aren't mobile, they don't pick up a lot of dirt; and aside from the inevitable spit up and poop, they should remain relatively clean unless you're swaddling them in rags from the garage (which—don't). When the time comes for baby's first tub (or sink) bath, you'll want to keep these things in mind.

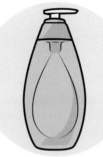

Be sure to use baby shampoo and soap that won't burn the eyes.

Gently wash baby with warm water and a soft cloth. Remember, baby's skin is ultra sensitive. Even a coarse cloth can be an irritant.

A tub lounger works well when baby is small, but be sure to have a side dish of warm water for cleaning.

LOOK OUT!
In addition to being on alert for incoming pee and poop, be aware of a sudsy baby's ability to jerk, squirm or punch you in the eye.

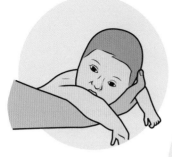

Before washing baby's bottom, first cradle their head and arms with one hand.

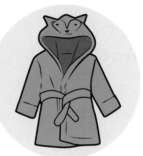

Have baby's bathrobe at the ready. Feel free to wear your own.

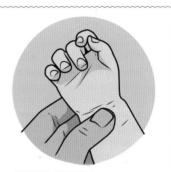

Make sure to clean thoroughly between the folds of skin, particularly on beefier babies. If their little creases and crevices go unwashed, the skin can become irritated and a painful red rash may develop in those spots.

TAKE EXTRA CARE WITH...

Nails
These are paper thin but can do some damage if not tended to. Keep them trimmed or filed so they don't get too long.

Genitalia
Both boys' and girls' genitalia need to be clean and free of any waste to prevent infection.

Belly button
Until it falls off, be very careful to keep the belly button scab dry, which will help it fall off. Don't try to remove it yoursel.

The First (For Them) Doctor's Appointment

By now, you're an old pro at the offices of your health care providers, be they pediatrician, OB-GYN, midwife, psychiatrist or otherwise. Your baby, on the other hand, is a straight up rookie: They have no idea what's going on. So it's your job to guide them through this strange experience. In your capacity as logistical wizard of the prenatal and postpartum worlds, you'll be relieved to note that this appointment will have been on the books since before you all were discharged from the hospital, so all you have to do is show up! And, er, don't forget Mom and your child when you do.

WHAT'LL HAPPEN
The doctor will do a physical examination of baby's general health, take notes on how they're growing (don't be alarmed if the baby's weight has gone down since birth: this is normal) and suggest any changes to make moving forward.

Be pepared!
Just like Scar says in a movie you're likely to watch repeatedly for several years: be prepared. Make sure baby is dressed in loose-fitting clothing and your diaper bag is packed in advance.

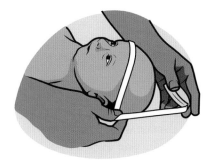

Baby's height and head circumference will be measured and recorded.

Ask questions

As many as you can think of. Don't be afraid to call with any questions you forget to ask in the office or think of after you leave.

Cover up

Your baby's immune system is very vulnerable. Make sure baby's bassinet or car seat is covered to keep germs away, especially in the waiting room.

Paperwork

Make sure your diaper bag has at least one extra pen. It's always better to use your own (see our note about baby's immune system) and make sure to bring your baby's important paperwork with you for your pediatrician's file.

Things you may be asked about...

Sleeping patterns (you and baby), digestion, feeding patterns, any irregularities in baby's eating and anything else you've noted.

Yes, you can swap your doc

Hey, no one is perfect, and if you and your pediatrician are no longer vibing, start shopping for a new caregiver. You're going to be spending a lot of time with this doctor, so make sure you can stand being in the same room with them.

Schedule the next appointment

Should be about a month from the first visit.

A NOTE ON VACCINES

It's important to have an honest conversation with your pediatrician. A lot of doctors won't take kids as patients if they don't follow the state's guidelines for vaccinations. Science has come a long way and doctors know best when it comes to your child's health. When you plan for your baby's vaccines, remember to make sure you and everyone who will be in close contact with your little one are fully vaccinated—flu shots, whooping cough, COVID-19, etc.

Baby Milestones

As your baby grows over the first few months of its life, you'll inevitably find yourself watching for markers of that growth. With equal parts excitement and apprehension, parents track every second as they witness their children develop in quantifiable ways, and all kinds of people have tried to attach "proper" timelines to these markers, everything from your kid recognizing your voice to speaking in full sentences. Do your best to be patient and celebrate each step while remembering that your kid is yours, but also an individual. Even though you or Mom may consider yourselves overachievers, your baby is on their own timeline. Unless your pediatrician has concerns, there is no correct time for any of these checkpoints to occur.

1. Voice recognition
During the first week, a newborn can recognize your voice, an important part of how baby learns to be comfortable in their environment. While they can't understand your words, don't let that discourage you from talking and singing to baby all day. If you're fluent in more than one language, use them all: You might think this baby talk is just nonsense, but you're doing important work toward building baby's language muscle.

2. Eye movement
After a few weeks, baby can likely see shapes about a foot in front of them, and will track the movement of your head and face. Try moving your head from side to side and see if their eyes follow you. This exercise can help build their eye dexterity and tracking skills.

WHAT BABY IS SEEING

From the time they are born, your baby's eyes are still coming into focus. Newborns cannot see very far, but as they grow, colors take shape and they can recognize toys, people and even themselves! It'll still be awhile before they can mow the lawn.

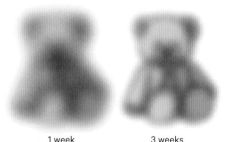

1 week   3 weeks

3. Stronger neck

You'll notice baby's neck getting stronger week by week, but you'll need to maintain constant support during this early period.

4. Cooing

At some point in the first couple of months, baby's vocal vocabulary will likely expand beyond just crying. Look for cooing, ahhs and baby's first attempts at mimicry. Don't worry—you've still got plenty of time before you institute a family swear jar.

5. Discovering their hands

At some point, your baby will discover their hands and all the fun digits that move independently. Allow them to experiment with these wonderful new discoveries by offering an assortment of toys with a variety of textures for them to touch and hold.

JEEPERS CREEPERS
Because they are not fully developed, you may see baby's peepers going in opposite directions as if they're a punch-drunk cartoon character. Don't be alarmed—this is normal.

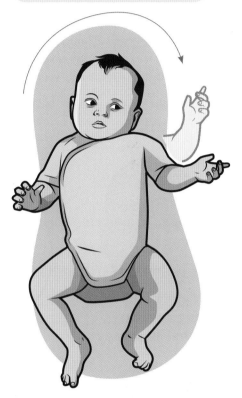

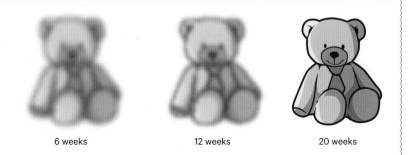

6 weeks   12 weeks   20 weeks

Funny Face-Off!

One of the most enjoyable parts of being a dad is playing games and goofing around with your kid. While it may take a few weeks for baby to have a reaction to your antics, it's well worth the wait once they crack a smile and recognize the funny man in front of them. There's no script for how to have fun with baby, but if you want some ideas to unleash your inner kid, here are some go-tos to get you started.

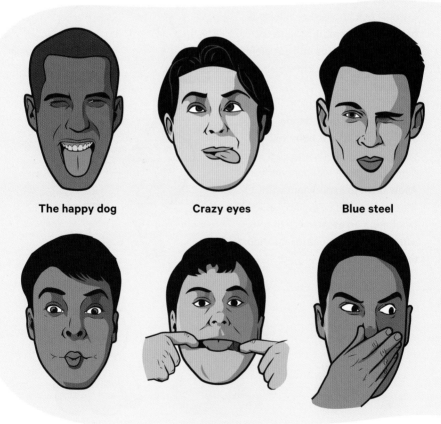

The happy dog

Crazy eyes

Blue steel

Fish face

Pulled cheeks

The stinky

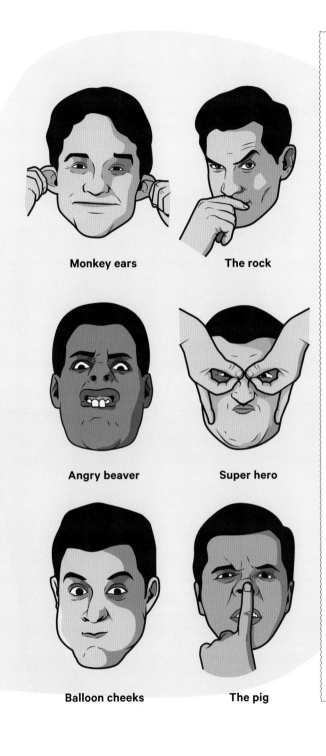

Monkey ears

The rock

Angry beaver

Super hero

Balloon cheeks

The pig

OPTIONS FOR WHEN YOUR FACE GETS TIRED FROM MUGGING

Sub in a stuffed animal
As much as your baby likes your face, they also love teddy bears, rabbits, dollies and any other friendly stuffed critter.

Change of scenery
Go outside or even just to another room to change up the environment. Babies love to explore and see new things.

Sing songs with action moments
"Ring Around the Rosie," "Itsy Bitsy Spider" and other nursery rhymes are popular because they have actions associated with the song (i.e., falling down, making a crawling spider with your hand). Babies love this extra layer of engagement. So put down your phone.

Read to baby
Even though they can't read or understand you, associating the story with the visuals in a book is essential for communication development. Reading is, as they say, fundamental.

Rib
Just what it sounds like. These marbled, tender cuts from the cow's upper midsection include rib-eye steak, rib roast (aka prime rib) and short ribs.

How to Know Your Beef Cuts

As a dad, you might be expected to be the grillmaster-in-chief. And before you can serve up burgers and steaks that'll make your family proud, you've got to learn the fundamentals of all things beef. Here's how to know a cow from snout to tail.

1
Chuck
This meat is naturally tougher than most beef cuts because it's found in the neck and shoulder region, the first of the forequarter (or front half) of a cow. Break down that muscle by braising or roasting it—pop it in a slow cooker and simmer it low and slow until it falls apart with a fork.

2
Brisket
Whether you slice it thin and barbecue it Korean style, cure it to make pastrami or corned beef or smoke it for nearly a day in a savory dry rub, this classic cut comes from the breast area.

> **DID YOU KNOW?**
> About 64 percent of a cow is used for food, but the rest of the animal is used to make various products, including antifreeze, blood thinners, cosmetics, insulin, jet fuel and toothpaste.

3
Fore shank and rear shank
Like chuck meat, this comes from a high-muscle, low-fat area—in this case, the upper portion of the foreleg—so it yields the best results when braised. Or use it to make beef stock (or a killer boeuf bourguignon).

5
Short loin

Located at the beginning of the hindquarter or back half of a cow, this upper midsection area yields porterhouse steaks, T-bone steaks, filet mignon and strip steak. They're pricey, so don't mess these up! Pan sear or grill with care.

6
Sirloin

While this area doesn't have the marbling found in New York strip or rib-eye, sirloin steaks (flat bone/round bone), top sirloin steak and tri-tip roast all make for flavorful, ideal cuts of meat to throw on the grill, broil or even sous vide.

7
Round

The back end of the cow consists of the rump, the upper portion (rump roast, tip roast and tip steak) and the round lower portion (round roast and round steak). Not much marbling to be found here, so you'll want to stick to slow-cooking, use it to make burgers and sausages or thinly slice it and dry it for jerky.

8
Flank

This comes from the cow's abdominal area. Not as tender as the previously mentioned rib or short loin but delicious and lean when prepared with care. It's best when braised, broiled, pan-fried or marinated and grilled, and it's also far easier on your wallet than many cuts.

9
Short plate

Below the rib portion of a cow lies its stomach area, aka the short plate, from which we get skirt steak—think fajitas, stir-fry, churrasco, etc.

Other cuts include the tongue, heart, kidneys, liver, oxtail and sweetbreads (organ meat that can be grilled or braised).

Chapter 7

ALL ABOUT SLEEP

Everyone needs rest, but finding the time can be challenging for new parents. Make sure you and Mom are getting your Z's, and when your baby is ready, sleep training will get them snoozing through the night. Buckle up.

Sleep: Mom First, Then Dad

The Sandman is a tough creditor, and any debts we accrue must be paid. When we don't get enough sleep, our brains can't recharge, which prevents us from functioning like normal, non-feral human beings. Science (and anecdotal experience) has proven a lack of sleep makes us more susceptible to illness and irritability, which are serious detriments when your primary objective is caring for a helpless infant. One of your many new jobs as Dad is to ensure everyone gets the rest they need.

If Mom is breastfeeding, it's going to be a lot easier for you to catch some winks than it will be for her, since only one of you is a 24/7 milk bar. If Mom's not getting enough sleep, you'll need to step up to the plate and manage baby's needs to give her ample time to recharge. The days of getting a solid eight hours of uninterrupted sleep (if they ever existed) will remain out of reach for quite some time, which means you'll have to make the most of what you can get. Follow these steps to get Mom, baby and eventually you into a good sleep routine

1. Follow baby's rhythm

Babies love routine. In these early months, they're the ones running the show. Conform to the rhythm that works for them and try to stick to it.

2. Take turns on the graveyard shift

Late-night feedings are tough, so make sure to share the burden. Dad should keep the milk or formula stocked and have bottles ready to go.

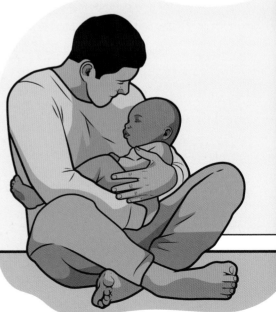

FORTRESS OF SOLITUDE

It's not a bad idea to sleep in different rooms to get more productive rest, especially if that room is devoid of a crying baby. Like Superman, you'll need to recharge before saving the planet. Don't worry—this arrangement won't last forever.

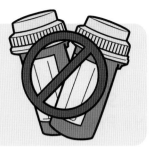

AVOID SLEEP MEDS

Most sleep medications warn not to operate heavy machinery after dosing, and your baby is more complicated than a Bobcat. You don't want to feel out of it if your kid needs you, so unless your doc says otherwise, leave any drowsiness-inducing meds on the shelf. If you can't, make a plan.

3. Set the scene

Mom, Dad and baby all need a calming, dark environment for sleep. Make sure your spaces are soothing, noise consistent, welcoming and dimly lit. That said, if you drift off in your living room watching anime that's fine too.

4. Accept help

There are no awards for functioning without sleep, only demerits. If you can't catch up on rest, ask for help. Grandparents, family and friends all want to be of assistance, so take them up on their offers so you can steal away for some shut-eye.

5. When in doubt, write It down

You think you'll remember but you won't. A lack of sleep kills our recall, so it helps to keep a notepad (or notes app) at the ready to jot down important info like when the baby last ate, what groceries you're running low on, upcoming appointments, etc. Life might feel like a test sometimes, but it's still open book. Use your notes. Future You sends his thanks in advance.

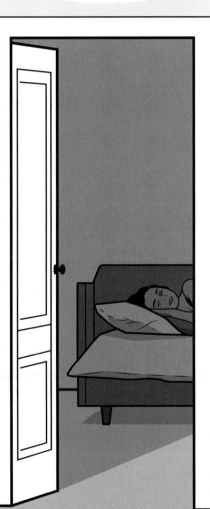

No Sleep? No Problem

Part of being a dad is adjusting to an unpredictable sleep schedule. Being alert is essential with a newborn (who can be unpredictable, to say the least), and mastering some crucial tricks can make the difference between high functioning and non-functioning. If you're finding it difficult to stand at attention on active dad duty, try these techniques from Billy Jensen and Check Freedman, coauthors of *Survival Ready: Life-Saving Skills and Expert Advice for Surviving Any Threat at Any Time.*

1. Get chatty
Though you're probably craving peace and quiet, a tranquil environment is risky as it could lull you to sleep. Instead of silently sinking into the couch as you keep an eye on your kid, talk to someone, whether it's your spouse/partner or a friend on the phone. Active conversation can be key to staying awake.

2. Water wake-up
Whether you're drinking it or bathing in it, water is one of the most effective energy sources around. If you're able, take a cold shower the morning after a sleepless night to jolt yourself awake. While you're on Dad duty, keep chugging H_2O—if you hydrate to the point where you require frequent trips to the restroom, you'll be very alert (as well as very hydrated).

3. Step Into the sunlight
The sun is notorious for waking you up in the morning, which means it can also be used to keep you awake throughout the day. If you're feeling groggy on a sunny day, use that natural light to your advantage: step outside for about five to 10 minutes and periodically close your eyes and turn your face toward the sun. Those warm rays will reset your internal clock and leave you feeling refreshed.

4. Make some moves
Exercise can give you a needed energy boost, but you'll of course need to be careful not to exhaust yourself even further. Try a session of simple squats, jumping jacks or simply go up and down the stairs in your house a handful of times. Once you increase your blood flow, you'll begin to feel more energized.

5. Fuel up with food
Coffee and energy drinks aren't always the best choices for keeping you on your toes. There are plenty of foods with the right nutrients to keep you awake and alert, such as cheese, chickpeas, almonds, peanuts, pumpkin seeds, tuna, edamame and hard-boiled eggs.

DON'T OVERDO IT
The ability to function on very little sleep is in the new dad job description, but true exhaustion is dangerous for both you and baby. If you're struggling to remember simple info, experiencing mood swings or losing motor coordination, call for backup.

HOW TO
CLEAR YOUR MIND

Even if you can't take an actual nap during the day, you can still give your brain a break. The art of daily meditation isn't always easy, but once you pull it off, you'll feel refreshed and ready to regain focus.

1. Have a designated space for mind-clearing.

2. Focus on your breathing.

3. Remove reminders of time from the area (calendars, clocks, your watch, etc.)

4. Comfort is key: A cushy couch or chair will help you relax (just don't lie down on a bed).

5. Prepare in advance: If possible, avoid stressful discussions in the hours beforehand.

6. Allow your mind to wander. Let thoughts pass through you like waves of water.

7. Queue up some soothing music or white noise (but then keep screens well out of reach).

8. When you're ready to end a session, slowly open your eyes and take notice of your surroundings.

Sleep Aids

Check out these low- and high-tech ways for your baby to catch some Z's.

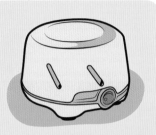

THE HOLY GRAIL
A white noise machine drowns out unwanted noise and can help baby stay asleep longer.

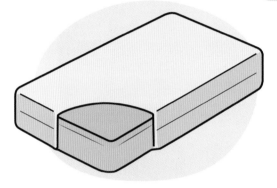

Breathable mattress
Typically designed with a porous surface, this ensures that baby will have no problem breathing if they roll over onto their stomach.

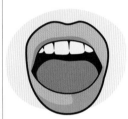

Your voice
Your baby associates your voice with comfort—humming, singing, talking in soothing tones or shushing can do the trick.

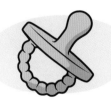

Pacifier
You might decide that you don't want your baby to have the option of a pacifier. You might also change your mind, so it's good to have a few on hand just in case.

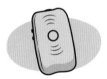

Baby calmer
Place this handy gadget close to baby's ear and allow the soothing sounds to lull them to sleep (just check the volume first).

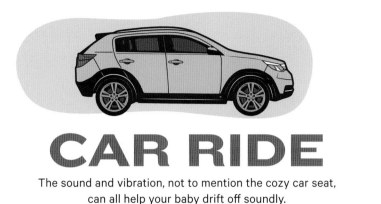

CAR RIDE

The sound and vibration, not to mention the cozy car seat,
can all help your baby drift off soundly.

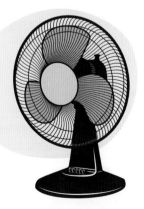

Music and light machine

Think Pink Floyd laser light show at the
local planetarium, but for babies. See
you on the dark side of your eyelids.

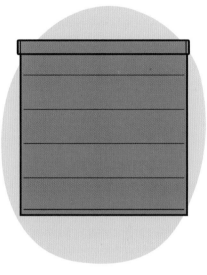

Blackout curtains

Setting the stage for bedtime and naps is
critical. If you have a sunny room, be sure to
have the ability to darken the light midday.

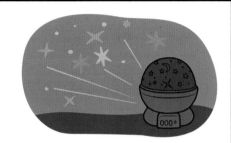

Your Dad's old fan

A classic sleep-soother that provides
the hum and the breeze all at once.

TOO-RA-LOO-RA-LOO-RAL

Singing a lullaby is an age-old trick that
babies love. Can't remember one or don't
know any? Check out "Too-Ra-Loo-Ra-
Loo-Ral (That's an Irish Lullaby)" by Bing
Crosby and give it a whirl. It's a classic
and easy to learn. Make up your own
lyrics or sing in step with Bing; either
way, your baby will love it.

Sleep Training

The first morning you wake up and realize your kid slept through the night without crying is a glorious one, and should be celebrated—it is the beginning of a new era for Mom and Dad. But you won't get there without some effort. There have been entire books written on the subject of getting your baby to fall asleep, and you will undoubtedly hear friends and family tell of their own journeys.

Take every bit of advice with a grain of salt (even what follows here) because your baby is yours, and might not be the same as Judy and Greg's. The most important thing to do is stick with what works. Parents should do what they feel comfortable doing, and if you need help, don't be afraid to ask for it from an expert. There are a number of methods that have worked over time and continue to be successful for parents and babies: Your consultation will likely include a discussion of at least one of the following methods.

Cry it out (CIO)

Popular, firmly established, but definitely not for everyone. The plan? Put baby safely in the crib once they've been fed, and—even if they're still awake—leave them there until they fall asleep. This is tough, because they will most likely cry (a lot). It's often harder on Mom and Dad than the baby, but if you choose this method, remember there are other things that they might be upset about besides separation anxiety, like a messy diaper or stuck leg, that require frequent check-ins.

Why It Works: It's tough love for sure, but if your baby has a full belly and they are tired, they'll eventually fall asleep.

The Ferber Method

Created by Dr. Richard Ferber, this classic plan for sleep training involves gradually breaking

---

BE COOL, DUDERINO

Sure, you can go into sleep training like a military drill sergeant and probably get results, but it's going to be hard on you, and not a lot of fun. If they're not ready to sleep through the night, be a bit more patient: The time will come.

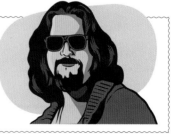

THE SHHHHHH

Self-explanatory: The calming powers of this simple sound are ancient. It ain't broke, so don't fix it. Just don't overuse it.

BACK RUBS

Physical contact is key for comfort—that's why it's one of the first things babies get after being born. Deliver the goods!

A FUN GAME

If you don't teach them early, you'll never feel the pride of the first time your kid beats you at your favorite game. Start with peek-a-boo. Save Texas hold 'em for when they have an allowance.

A ROUTINE

Think of putting your baby to sleep like an existential foul shot or golf swing: The key to success is muscle memory; doing the same exact thing every single time. Eventually, bedtime will be practically coded into them.

SINGING A LULLABY

And it doesn't have to be from the public domain, either: lullaby-ify your favorite pop tunes and give baby a sense of the good stuff early.

PATIENCE

After spending most of their time in Mom's uterus and being cuddled non-stop shortly after birth, babies are accustomed to the feeling of a parent close to them. Loosening that expectation will take a bit, but don't lose heart. You'll have your eight hours again soon.

SUPPORT

It's good to lean on your partner during this time, but if you need additional help, call friends, family or your doctor to guide you through the ups and downs of sleep training.

Sleep Training

(CONTINUED)

your baby's need to be held and comforted over time. Put your baby in their crib once the nighttime routine is over. When baby wakes, rub their back or comfort them gently until they fall back asleep. When they wake again, wait a little longer before entering their room and offering comfort. Over time, baby will need less support until they are sleeping through the night and dreaming about their independence.

Why It Works: It's gradual enough that baby has time to develop some self-soothing techniques.

Night weaning

Night weaning is making sure your baby is eating their meals during the day so they don't wake up craving a fourth meal at 3 a.m., but it also impacts sleep training. Think of it as introducing a normal schedule gradually and letting baby's eating schedule dictate their

sleep. This will likely necessitate another method like CIO to drive the point home should your baby wake up in the night despite their large dinner.

Why It Works: By feeding baby one large meal before bed, they'll have plenty of sustenance to get them through the night. As you train with baby, their stomach grows, as will their familiarity with sleeping at a specific time.

The chair method

Also known as the stool method (but since your whole world is poop right now, Chair Method sounds less scatological), this involves some type of seat for you or Mom (pick a comfy one because the rest of this process is… uncomfortable). It's similar to the Ferber Method in that it involves a gradual movement to a normal schedule, but in this case, you're the one doing the gradual moves, not the baby. When your baby is drowsy, put them in a crib, then sit in a chair next to them. Once they fall asleep, leave the room. If they begin to cry, come back to your chair. Every few nights, move the chair back a few feet until you're eventually out of the room. This method can be tough on the parent

> **SAFETY FIRST**
> Don't put anything in the crib that could be a choking hazard, including blankets, toys and bottles. Nothing should dangle into the crib either.

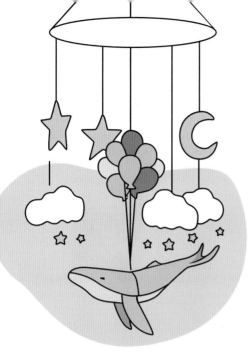

TRUST YOUR INSTINCTS

Sleep training is difficult, and no matter which method (or combo of methods) you choose, you will undoubtedly have setbacks and frustration. If you think something isn't working, don't do it. Eventually, it'll all click and a sleep-filled night for all will become your new normal.

(especially if baby gets fussy) since you're meant to sit there until baby racks out. And it may be confusing for the baby to see you but not feel your loving embrace no matter how hard they cry. It's not as hardcore as the CIO method, but it still takes a fair amount of willpower.

Why It Works: This lighter version of the CIO method is a tough-love way of helping baby understand, "Everything is OK. It's safe to sleep now. One day you too will have a favorite chair."

Bedtime fading

This isn't sleep training so much as a method to manipulate baby's sense of time. For example, if you typically put them down around 7 p.m. but they cry for about 30 minutes in their crib, their natural bedtime (aka the one corresponding to their circadian rhythm) is likely closer to 7:30 p.m. You can move bedtime back to match that rhythm by delaying it a few more minutes each night.

Why It Works: Knowing your baby's natural sleep patterns is half the battle. The other half is putting that knowledge to use, likely by applying one of these other methods.

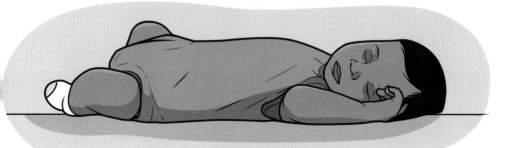

How to Split Firewood and Make a Fire

A family camping trip is a rite of passage once you become a dad; and if all goes well, it can even become a tradition. To make sure no one gets left out in the cold, here's how you can make a classic campfire.

BEFORE YOU BEGIN

Keep a shovel and a bucket of water at the ready in case you make too good of a fire and have to throw dirt or H_2O on it. And of course, make sure Mom or another adult is keeping an extra close eye on your kid throughout the process.

LOOK THE PART

If you're out in the wild, dress appropriately. You can't go wrong with a comfortable flannel, boots, jeans and a vest. A beard is optional, but encouraged.

(1)

Gather good wood

Small, dry logs make the best campfire fuel, but be sure to gather plenty of kindling (small sticks) and tinder (wood shavings, twigs, dry grass and leaves) as well. Don't worry about overstocking—you always want extra wood handy to keep the fire going as long as desired.

(2)

Start splitting

Set the log vertically on flat ground. Swing your axe downward so the thin edge of the blade goes into the top surface of the log. With enough dad-power, the log should split into two fairly even halves. Repeat this process until you have a nice pile of logs ready to be fed to your fire.

(3)

Pick your spot

Find a clear, dry area on the ground where the wind won't interfere with your flames. Make sure you're at least 6 feet away from any bushes, trees and grass.

(4)

Light it up

In the spot you've chosen for the fire, stack your kindling in a crisscross or tepee shape, then place your tinder in between and around the kindling. Light the tinder with a match or lighter. Once it begins to burn and the fire grows, add more tinder and blow on the base of the flames. Add a little more kindling, then add some of those logs you expertly chopped.

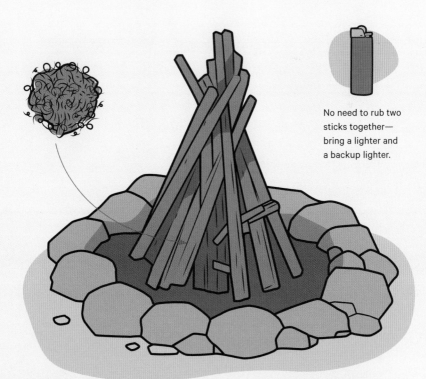

No need to rub two sticks together— bring a lighter and a backup lighter.

Chapter 8

3-9 MONTHS OLD

Just when you've figured out how to take care of a baby, they turn into a tot. After you mastered bottle feeding, they've sprouted a tooth and are chowing down on pureed carrots. It's been said "they grow up fast," and while the days may seem long, your child is growing like a weed and will never be this small again. Here's how to make the most of that time.

How to Pack a Diaper Bag

The diaper bag travels with you wherever you go. While its chief purpose is to store all the essentials for on-the-go diaper changes, it also primes your baby for almost every scenario and gives you a chance to show off your preparedness skills.

Organize the bag according to necessity. Changing pad, diapers and wipes should be the easiest to access, followed by pacifiers and baby bottles, then the least-used items—e.g., Band-aids.

1

Diapers

A top priority item (see pg. 126). Store these in an easy-to-reach spot.

2

Wipes

Pack travel-sized wipes next to diapers and the changing pad.

3

Changing pad

Some bags come with one included, but check the size—you may need a larger one.

4

Baby cream

Essentials for diaper changes. Choose a small tube to save space.

5

Small waste bags

For soiled diapers and other trash.

6

Pacifiers

Keep one or three of these self-soothers in a side pocket for easy access.

7

Hand sanitizer

Because germs are everywhere and things get gross fast.

8

Food for baby

Formula, breast milk, crackers—whatever your little one eats, carry some with you all the time.

9

Change of clothes

In case there's an unexpected blowout or messy meal or their friend shows up for a playdate in the same onesie.

10

Small toys

It's nice to have some distraction items in case of an emergency.

WHAT NOT TO PACK

It might be tricky to judge the essentials from any possible scenario, but avoid packing large bulky items and anything that you don't use on a regular basis like cough syrup, aquatic diapers or extra shoes.

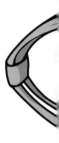

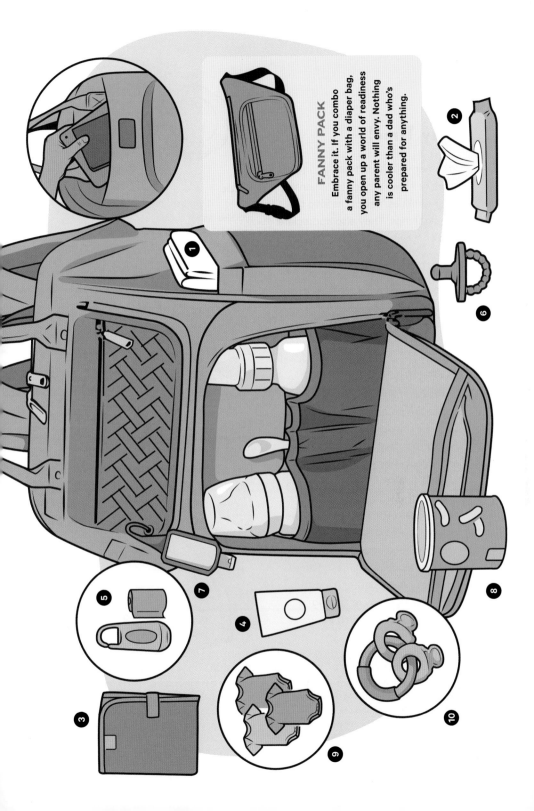

FANNY PACK

Embrace it. If you combo a fanny pack with a diaper bag, you open up a world of readiness any parent will envy. Nothing is cooler than a dad who's prepared for anything.

Play Time!

Whether you tickle them, snuggle them or snuggle them or blow raspberries against their tummies, newborns love the simple things. They also appreciate nursery rhymes that involve actions or sounds, like "Itsy Bitsy Spider" (see pg. 190).

You will undoubtedly have many toys ready for your kid to play with, but it's a good idea to slowly introduce them to toys one by one rather than all at once (lest you risk blowing their tiny minds).

Toys that light up or make noises are popular with newborns because they engage their senses. Babies also love different textures and discovering if an action has a result. Cause and effect is a concept they'll love to learn. If they push a button on the farm toy, the cow moos—huzzah!

But you don't need to buy the fanciest, loudest, whirliest gizmos. Just have fun, whether it's with a store-bought toy or the big cardboard box it arrived in.

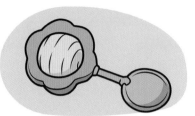

Rattle
A tried and true baby toy: It's colorful and provides instant auditory satisfaction upon shaking. Embrace this simple pleasure.

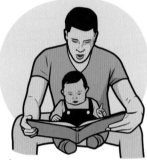

Books
Embedding books, language and the habit of reading into your child is a smart move. Start 'em early and read to them as much as you can.

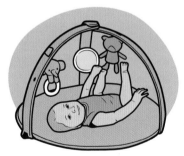

Play mat
The play mat can be a win-win for baby and parent. Dangling engagement can provide loads of entertainment that benefits development and hand-eye coordination.

SAFETY FIRST
Many toys that look kid-friendly aren't meant for newborns. Read the indicated age range and use common sense. If it's complex or has small pieces, save it for when they're older.

TUMMY TIME

It's not all fun and games when having fun and...uh...playing games. Tummy time is an essential part of strengthening your baby's core and getting their muscles strong to support their heads and body. Don't skip it.

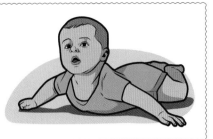

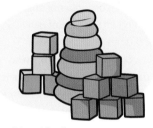

Battery powered gizmo
A toy that lights up and makes noise is good for baby to experience in small doses. It's good for sensory development and your little one will love it.

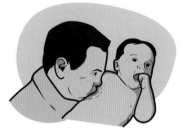

Stacking blocks
Stacking blocks is rewarding. Smashing those blocks down is a blast! Repeat until exhausted.

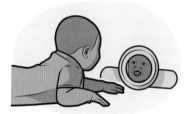

Mirrors
Need a break? Introduce your baby to themselves. There's a chance they'll hit it off and entertain each other for an hour.

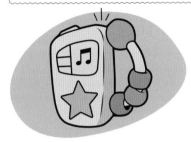

Raspberries
Not the fruit—the hilarious mouth-on-tummy fart blow every kid loves.

PEEK-A-BOO

When your baby reacts to playing peek-a-boo, get the camera and record that moment of pure joy. Hiding your face then reappearing is a magic trick that amazes even the most critical of babies, since they haven't yet learned about object permanence.

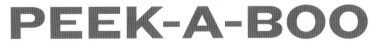

Sex After Baby

It's generally recommended that a woman wait four to six weeks after having a baby to resume having sex. This can be longer or shorter depending on the type of delivery, healing times and many other factors. Since Mom's the one who had the baby, this timeline works in accordance with her health. If she's not ready, then neither are you, cowboy. Just know that physical intimacy is, by definition, unique to you and your partner. Do what works for you. Here are some common questions you may want to consider.

1. Does it hurt?
If Mom gave birth vaginally, sex can definitely be painful. Use lube, go slow and if it's too uncomfortable, stop, wait another week or so and try again later.

2. What if Mom had a Cesarean birth?
While your partner's vagina doesn't have to heal, the incision on her stomach will. A C-section is major surgery and she likely won't enjoy pressure on her tummy. Shag accordingly.

3. Should we use birth control?
Some believe Mom can't get pregnant while she's breastfeeding or before her period reappears. And they are absolutely wrong. A woman can get pregnant just weeks after giving birth, so use caution if you're not ready to flip back to Chapter 1 before your

> **EMBRACING INTIMACY**
> You've got a full plate: Mom's body has its share of healing to do and your new roommate is needy, to say the least. Remember: Being intimate with your partner isn't limited to penetrative sex (as an example, no new mother has ever refused a foot massage).

kid's first birthday. The Mayo Clinic advises parents wait 18 months before trying for a second child—having a baby sooner means increased risk of premature birth, congenital disorders and other health problems.

4. Does it always have to be a quickie? What if they hear us?
If you and your partner are ready to have sex, you should make time for it when you can since the moment you get horizontal on a bed one of you is liable to pass out. Take the time you have however you like. Baby monitor technology has come a long way, so you can keep an eye on baby even while you're, um, preoccupied. As far as noise goes, your baby is unlikely to connect any sound you make during sex to the act itself. This is a fear you can set aside until they are older and more inclined to wander into your bedroom because they had a nightmare about howling monkeys.

5. What about low libido?
Mom's libido can fluctuate as her hormones change after delivery, and given the stresses of having a brand new tiny human to care for 24/7, you might find you aren't in the mood as often as you once were. This is normal—just keep the lines of communication open about how you're feeling and meet each other's needs in every way you can. If low libido persists, talk to your doctor or therapist about possible causes and potential solutions.

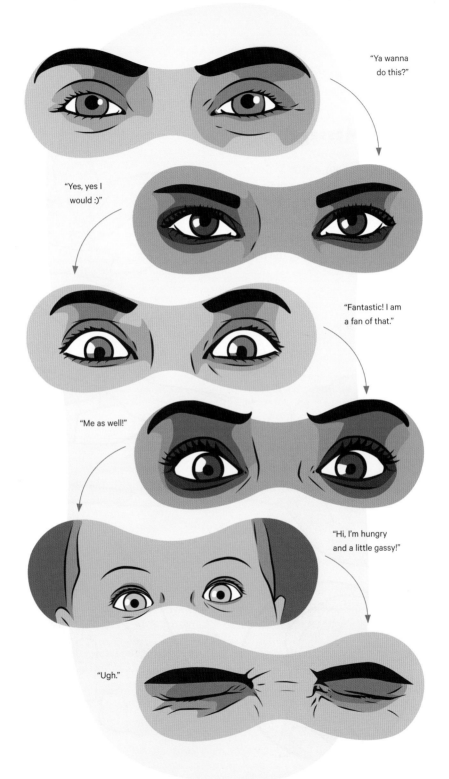

Baby Massage

Giving your baby a little TLC is a great way to moisturize their skin, check their reflexes and look for rashes. Here are some techniques you can employ to treat them to a spa day without leaving the house.

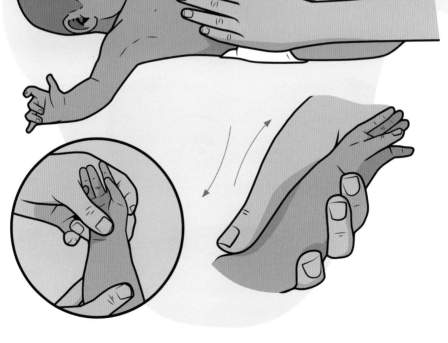

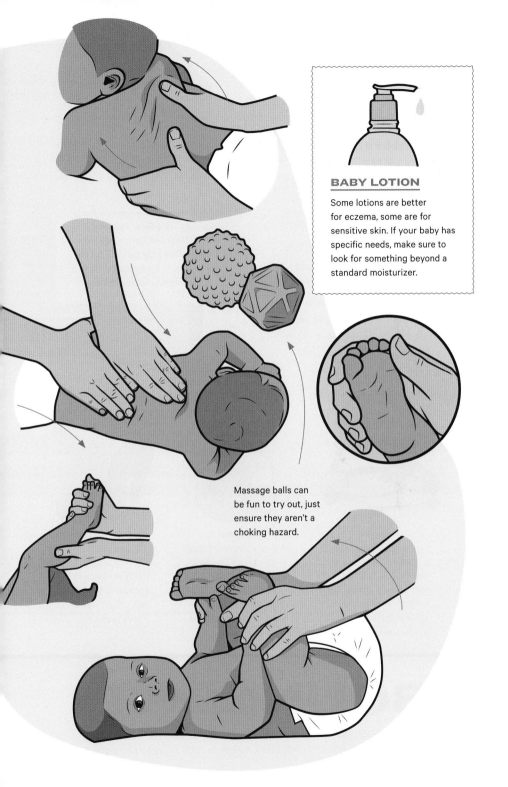

BABY LOTION

Some lotions are better
for eczema, some are for
sensitive skin. If your baby has
specific needs, make sure to
look for something beyond a
standard moisturizer.

Massage balls can
be fun to try out, just
ensure they aren't a
choking hazard.

Baby Movers and Stabilizers

Once your kid starts rolling over, they'll want to keep moving, and don't be surprised when they speed up with every turn. You'll want to encourage this, but also contain it ("Where's the baby?" is not a fun game, and heart attacks are still one of the leading causes of death among dads). Here's how to (ethically) lock them up and keep them from falling down.

PACK 'N PLAY

Maybe this classic becomes a staple of your living room, maybe it's strictly for travel, but Ye Olde Pack 'n Play will be a big part of your life for awhile. As such, you'll want to get one that unfolds with ease.

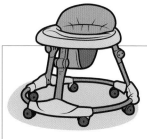

Coasters

These are a great way for baby to explore safely around your home (just don't let them wander out of sight). They're fun, and you'll probably wish you had one as well.

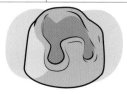

Bumbo

A Bumbo is a stable seat made of foam into which baby can fit snugly. It's safe for baby and perfect for parents who need to use both hands for a while.

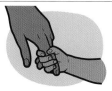

Dad's (or Mom's) finger

The best stabilizer on the market, and guaranteed to help your tot get where they're going.

BOUNCERS

Baby bouncers can provide a safe spot for baby and parent. And if you're lucky, the rhythmic bouncing could be enough to rock baby to sleepytown.

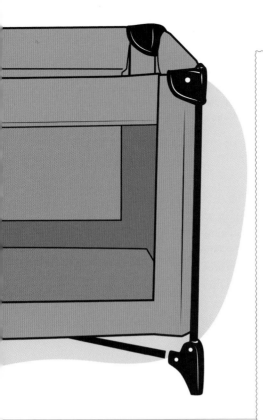

The second your kid starts moving, you're going to want to take safety measures to make sure they don't hurt themselves on stairs or sneak off to places they shouldn't. Different staircases and entryways will require specific installation that might necessitate a degree of customization. Be sure to measure the spaces involved carefully so the gates you choose fit snugly.

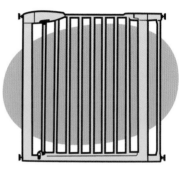

There are a number of different options when it comes to materials, closure type, height and other variables. Remember, you'll likely be opening and closing this gate with one hand, so make sure you're comfortable with the height and closure system you choose to prevent frustration later on. Be sure to read the instructions carefully, especially when attaching the gate to a banister

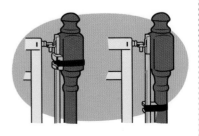

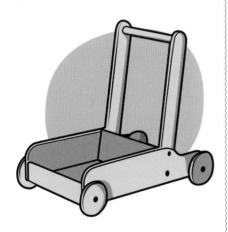

Walkers

They come in a variety of shapes and sizes, but they all basically act as a stepping stone (pun definitely intended) to baby walking on their own.

WHEN TO WORRY

If your baby is very fussy, has blood in their stool or is vomiting, contact a doctor right away. They may have an impaction, or something more serious than just gas.

How to Get Gas Out of Your Baby

Babies can be quite gassy, and a fart, while funny, is also a sign of healthy digestion. But what happens when the air gets stuck? There are some steps you can take to help your progeny get the gas out and prevent it from causing future discomfort. As your baby's digestive tract grows, the gas will become less of a problem for both of you. Till then, here's what you should know and how you can help.

What causes gas?

1. Gulping air while eating food (breast and bottle alike)
2. Sucking a pacifier
3. Crying
4. Foods like broccoli, beans, pears and milk

Signs to watch for:

1. Bloating
2. Burping
3. Crying
4. Farting
5. Hard tummy
6. Over-fussiness

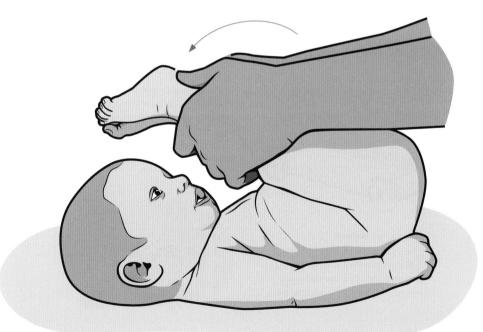

How to prevent gas

1. Check your feeding position

When bottle-feeding, keep the baby's head higher than their stomach. Due to gravity, the milk sinks to the bottom of the stomach while the air in the bottle stays at the top, away from baby's intake. Try tipping the bottle up slightly so there are no air bubbles in the nipple and use a pillow for support if needed.

2. Swap equipment

Use a slower flow nipple or try out a different bottle type designed to reduce gas.

3. Don't forget to burp

Burping your baby after every meal is a fairly essential step until your kid can manage this on their own.

A HELPFUL TOOL

Handy gadgets such as the Windi by Frida are simple but effective tools to alleviate baby's discomfort. If your tot is habitually gassy, you might want to stock up on these and use them as needed.

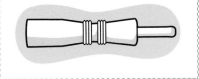

If no burp will come, let your baby rest for a few minutes, then try gently patting their back again.

4. Work it out

With your baby lying on their back, pump their legs back and forth as though they're pedaling a bike or give them tummy time (watch them while they lie on their stomach). A warm bath can also help relax their muscles.

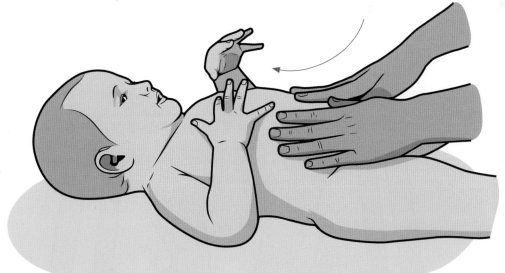

Introducing Solids

Once a baby begins to eat real food, experiencing various flavors and textures for the first time, it's pretty funny. It's also messy as hell. After a few practice flights, baby will get the hang of it and should be ready for a few rounds of Here Comes the Airplane. Start with

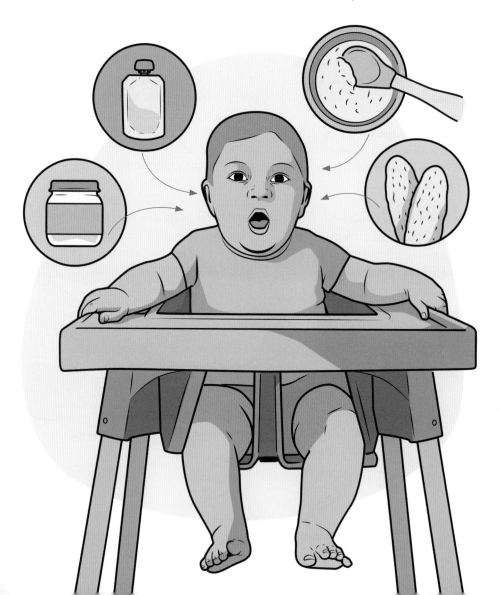

some type of mashed or pureed foods with a smooth texture: These have a close consistency to milk or formula and don't pose any choking hazards. You can also introduce baby cereal that mushes quickly in their mouth. If you decide to make all your own food, cook it thoroughly so it's easy to smash with a fork. Slowly introduce new foods every few days and before you know it, they'll be the tiniest little gourmand on the block.

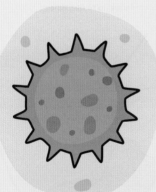

BE VIGILANT OF ALLERGIES

Potentially allergenic foods include cow's milk products, eggs, fish, shellfish, tree nuts, peanuts, wheat, soy and sesame. Talk with your pediatrician about how to safely introduce allergenic foods in case your baby has any adverse reactions.

KNOW YOUR NICKNAMES

When your kid starts chowing down on semi-real food, you may feel inclined to give them a nickname, if you haven't already. How do you know which name fits your kid? Give some a try and see how they (or Mom) react:

HOSS
Big, bold, authoritative

BUDDY
A happy baby who loves eating with others

CHUNK
A noticeably round child with rolls for days

PUDDIN'
Baby's got a sweet tooth

BUZZ
They love the airplane part of mealtime more than the food

DUKE/ DUCHESS
For discerning (read: fussy) eaters

SIR/MA'AM
The formality juxtaposes nicely with their total lack of self-awareness

LIL' MAN/MISS
A strong, independent baby who would rather feed themselves

SPORT
A baby inclined to play with their food

SQUIRT
They know what they did

What to Do If Baby Is Choking

CALL 911 IMMEDIATELY
Every second counts in an emergency. If someone else is around, have them call 911 while you work to dislodge the blockage. If you're alone and your actions aren't helping, call 911 for help.

The way babies test out something new is by putting it in their mouth. Anything smaller than 1¼ inches in diameter (e.g., marbles, bouncy balls, coins) is a choking hazard and should be removed from baby's environment. In fact, you'll begin removing any choking hazards from your life as the safe space in your home seemingly shrinks every day. As your child wanders the floors of your home, they will inevitably put something they absolutely should not in their mouth. Even food can be a hazard. If you see your baby choking, remain calm and get the blockage out as fast as possible.

1. Back blows

While supporting their head under the chin, hold baby facedown along your thigh with their head near your knee and their bottom near your waist. With the base of your palm, hit them firmly on the back between the shoulder blades up to five times.

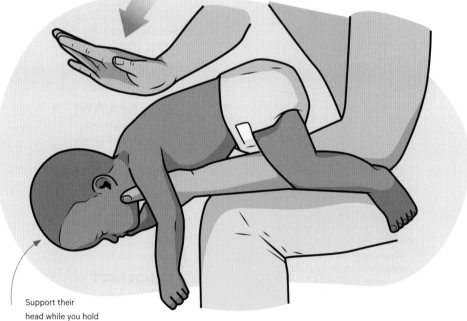

Support their head while you hold them in position

2. Chest thrusts

Turn baby over and place two fingers in the center of their chest just below the nipples. Push downward, sharply, up to five times. This should squeeze the air out of baby's lungs, which can dislodge the blockage.

3. Repeat

Continue with cycles of back blows and chest thrusts until the blockage dislodges, help arrives or the baby becomes unresponsive.

Removing from the mouth

If you cannot see the object in baby's throat, DO NOT attempt to remove it by reaching in their mouth, as this could cause further harm. Only attempt this if you can clearly see the blockage and can safely pluck it out with your fingertips.

JUST IN CASE...

If you want to be ready for any scenario, products such as a LifeVac or DeChoker can clear your baby's throat quickly. If you go this route, learn how to use these items and store them somewhere easily accessible.

Baby Babble

Babies develop communication skills faster when their parents respond with enthusiasm. If your kid points to their bottle and says "baba," repeat "baba," then say "bottle" with a big smile. The positive reinforcement will give your baby the confidence to try more sounds. Here are some more tips to get your kid chatting.

Name everything

Name things out loud as you show them to baby. If you're holding a toy duck, for example, say "Duck!" With repetition, your baby will begin to understand how to identify things.

Equate sounds to objects

Point to a toy car (or your vehicle) and say "Vroom, vroom!" This association helps your baby understand what sounds go with the objects they see.

PLAY THE REPEAT GAME

A fun way to get your kid talking is to imitate them as they imitate you. A good volley of words is very exciting for baby and repeating the same sound is great practice.

Ask questions

Try anything that's on your mind: "What color is the sky?" "Why is the house so hot?" "Do you think the Eagles will cover the spread?" Look directly at them, be animated with your face and voice, then follow up with an answer. Yes, you're talking to yourself, but you're modeling how a conversation (and also the world) works: "The sky is blue." "Because your mother is always cold but refuses to wear sweaters in July." "Yes, the Eagles cover because there is a God and he loves me."

Sing songs

A lot of baby songs are silly and full of outrageous antics, such as "Ring Around the Rosie." Everyone remembers the punch line "we all fall down" because it has a fun associated action, even if it is from a song about the bubonic plague.

Read books

Books are an excellent source of new words. Start with ones you remember from your childhood, then venture into others that might help them make conversational connections (e.g., books about dinosaurs if they have a favorite dinosaur toy).

UNDERSTANDING BABY BABBLE

Babies are lousy public speakers, but that doesn't stop them from trying. If baby points at something and makes a sound that's even vaguely similar to the word for that thing, chances are that's what they're talking about. Beyond that, who knows?!

Thwwwpffft!
"Had a piece of carrot stuck on my lip."

Baah-Bah
"Bottle me, bro."

Goo-Goo
"There may be a mess on the poop deck, sailor."

DaaDah!
"Dad!" or "Entertain me, clown!

GuhGUH!
"I have toys, where are they and why am I not holding one?

Maamuh!
"Mom!" or "My mutt" if you have a dog.

Ahhhbaat!
"Are you aware there's a bat in the attic?"

Dah!
"That thing right there!"

Kewkee?:
"Cookie. That wasn't a question."

More Baby Milestones

A lot of firsts can be expected to happen before baby is 9 months old. First time trying a lemon, playing in sand, maybe even a first step; it can all happen in the blink of an eye, so pay attention. Your pediatrician will be tracking these events closely to make sure the kid is hitting developmental markers as they grow. While every child is different, be sure to look out for the following:

Head support

After months of putting in long hours of tummy time, baby has developed strong neck muscles and can hold their own head up without toppling over. This is great for everyone because it means your baby's muscles are developing. But it doesn't mean you can leave them on their own quite yet.

Grasping

Mastering a new skill is very exciting for a baby. And when they figure out that they can control their hands and fingers, look out! They can grab hard and enjoy not letting go.

Teething

Typically, teeth appear as a little white dot and poke through the gums two at a time. This can cause sleep regression and be a little

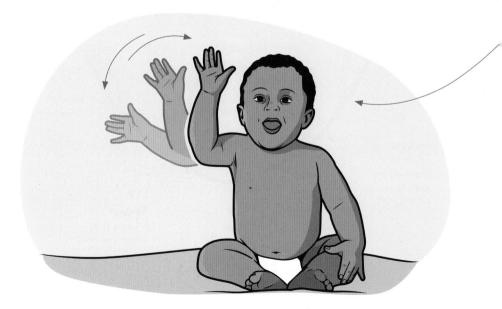

painful for your kid. Home remedies can help.

Self-soothing

If you've given your kid some space when they are crying, then you should notice some positive results during this period. They will learn how to self-soothe without Mom or Dad's help. Their first little step toward independence. Tear.

Waving hello and bye-bye

Calming their motor skills into a discernible action is a big event! Practice waving with your baby when entering or leaving a room, and your baby will soon pick up on salutation and make it a part of their daily life.

Interactive gaming

Once your kid gets the hang of how life works, and the comings and goings of your face, you can start to play games like peek-a-boo. Showing them something unexpected like a disappearing head is a guaranteed giggle-maker.

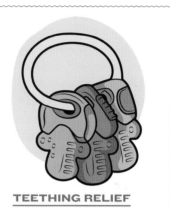

TEETHING RELIEF

Use these methods (not whiskey, it's not 1880) when your baby's chompers start poking through.

Teething toys
Too many shapes and sizes to list means you have plenty of options to choose from. Check your closets: You were probably gifted some of these before your baby was born.

Frozen washcloth
The cold acts as an immediate numbing agent, and the cloth is soft and fun to bite.

Chamomile
This natural remedy can soothe and relax your baby, making it a popular solve for parents.

Try rubbing your baby's gums
Wash your hands thoroughly or wet some gauze to rub your baby's gums. The pressure can ease your baby's discomfort.

How to Play Craps

Tossing your kid's college fund on red at the roulette table is a terrible idea for a number of reasons, only one of which is that you can get better odds playing craps. "Baby needs a new pair of shoes" is, for whatever reason, a classic exclamation when throwing dice at the craps table, and that's just one of several aspects of the game that can confuse those who have never played. But you're a dad now. Learning new things so you can pass them on to your kid is part of the gig (as is knowing that gambling can be fun but also addictive and is best done, like so many things, in moderation). Here's how to play.

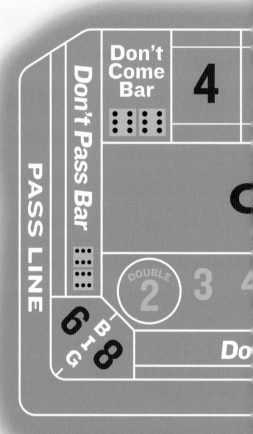

(1)

Start with a bet.
All craps games begin with a "pass line bet." Here, you bet that the dice will land on a 7 or 11 ("pass the line") or on a 2, 3 or 12 ("don't pass").

(2)

Roll the dice
The shooter will start the game with the first roll of the dice, known as the "come out roll."

(3)

Check your first bets.
If the dice land on 7 or 11 on the come out roll, pass line bets instantly win. "Don't pass bets" win if the dice land on a combined 2, 3 or 12. If the dice land on any other number, your pass line or don't pass bets remain in play for subsequent rolls.

(4)

Establish a point
Any other numbers (4, 5, 6, 8, 9 or 10) the dice lands on from the come out roll establish that number as the "point" on the craps table. Gameplay continues (as well as your pass line or don't pass bets) until the point number is rolled again or a 7 is rolled.

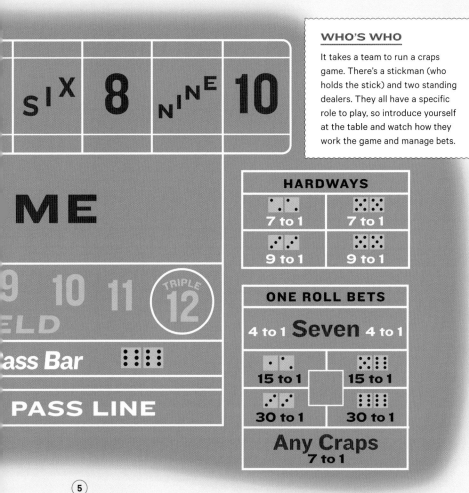

WHO'S WHO

It takes a team to run a craps game. There's a stickman (who holds the stick) and two standing dealers. They all have a specific role to play, so introduce yourself at the table and watch how they work the game and manage bets.

SIX **8** NINE **10**

ME

9 **10** **11** TRIPLE **12**

ELD

ass Bar

PASS LINE

HARDWAYS

7 to 1	7 to 1
9 to 1	9 to 1

ONE ROLL BETS

4 to 1 **Seven** 4 to 1

15 to 1	15 to 1
30 to 1	30 to 1

Any Craps
7 to 1

(5)

Add to your bets

Once a point has been set, you can then bet on the dice landing the point, landing on different numbers or losing completely by landing on 7. Six and 8 are a great place to start your wagering. You can also add to your pass line bet by asking for "odds," which allow you to make an informed bet to maximize your potential winnings.

(6)

Continue to shoot

The shooter will keep rolling the dice (and you can keep betting) until they land a 7 or the point.

(7)

End the round

If the point is rolled before a 7, all pass line bets will win. If a 7 is rolled before the point, all pass line bets will lose and all don't pass bets will win instead.

GOOD LUCK!

While these are just the basic rules, it's enough to get a spot at the table. Craps is a social game, so pay attention to the other players and how they bet and you'll be rolling like a pro in no time.

Chapter 9

YOUR BABY IS A YEAR OLD!

Congratulations, you've raised a kid for a year! What happens next is a continuation of what's been happening in your life already, with a few key differences. Baby is moving, and fast. They're also teething, talking, curious and probably getting a little temperamental. The game has changed, but the goal remains the same: Be the best dad possible.

Air Travel With a Kid

Taking your kid on a plane can be a stressful experience, but if you've prepared for the typical scenarios, it should be a relatively smooth flight from takeoff to touchdown.

Travel light

Pack as little as possible. You'll be carrying extra gear, which will typically include a car seat, stroller, pack 'n play and their clothes.

Get comfy

Wear comfortable clothing (always a good air travel tip) and shoes

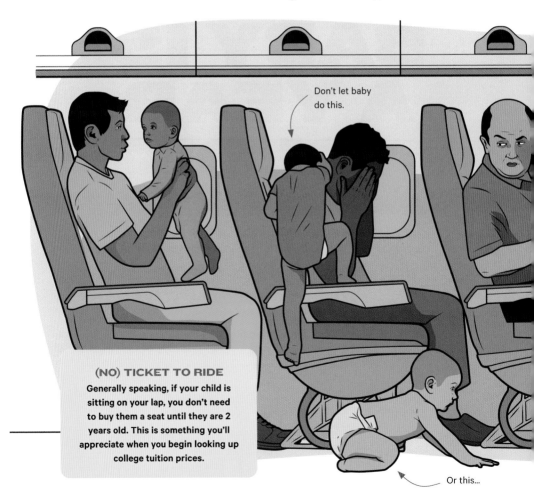

Don't let baby do this.

(NO) TICKET TO RIDE

Generally speaking, if your child is sitting on your lap, you don't need to buy them a seat until they are 2 years old. This is something you'll appreciate when you begin looking up college tuition prices.

Or this...

that are easy to slip in and out of. This goes a long way in reducing your stress levels.

Window or aisle

The window can provide entertaining views, while the aisle is good for easy bathroom access and moving around the cabin.

Don't sweat other people

You can't control how other people feel about traveling with a baby, so try not to worry about it. People either understand your challenges or they don't pity helpless babies. That said, feel free to go the extra mile and have ear plugs on hand if anyone would like them.

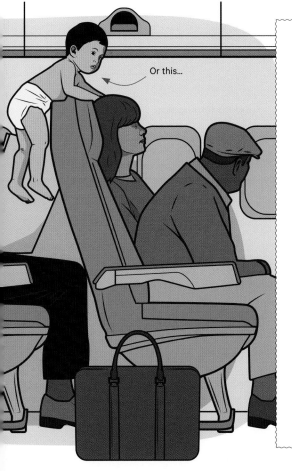

Or this...

MUST-HAVE TRAVEL CHECKLIST

To ensure a successful trip, be prepared for a variety of scenarios and have the following items at the ready:

✓ **Your child's birth certificate, passport and medical records**

✓ **Car seat and car seat cover for checking and storage**

✓ **A variety of snacks (for everyone)**

✓ **Sippy cup and bottle of milk or formula**

✓ **Sanitizing wipes. Germs are everywhere on a plane and your kid will try to put their mouth on everything, so clean the seats as soon as you sit down.**

✓ **Two or three toys. No need to bring the whole playroom, just a few fan favorites for easy entertainment.**

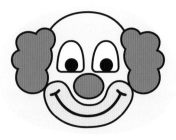

Eating in a Restaurant

Eventually, you're going to want to take the new tribe out for lunch or dinner, and you should! No need to make this a stressful event, just plan ahead. Make sure you're ready for some common scenarios and have the solution to keep your kid happy and relatively quiet for the whole meal.

Keep it kid-friendly

Many restaurants cater to families, but some don't. Make sure you're not trying to squeeze your stroller into that trendy new 10-seat speakeasy. And if you're not sure what the situation is, simple: Call the establishment beforehand.

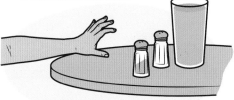

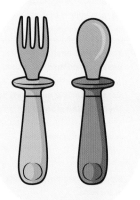

Set up for success

Kids like to grab everything in front of them. So as you take your seats, take account of what is within grabbing distance. Move everything out of your kid's reach, including utensils, salt and pepper, sugar packets and water glasses.

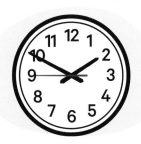

PRACTICE AT HOME

The best way to ensure a successful outing is good practice at home. Give your child an introduction to the dining experience and prep them with the basics of ordering, waiting and then enjoying a meal together.

Know your schedule

If your kiddo has a daily nap at 1 p.m., avoid that time at all costs. Ideally you would want to visit a restaurant after nap time or early in their usual meal window.

Most likely, the staff will be very accommodating to you and your family. Don't forget that when it comes time to add gratuity. Especially if you've made a mess.

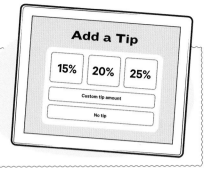

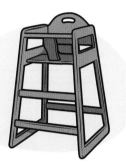

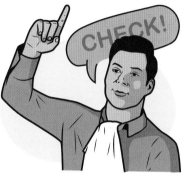

Keep them safe and secure

The restaurant may provide you with a high chair, but it's your job as Dad to make sure that what you are given is acceptable for your kid. Make sure the chair or booster is sturdy, secure and the right size for your child before putting them in.

Ask for the check early

You never know when your dining experience might go sideways thanks to your child's mood swings. Err on the side of caution and get the check soon after ordering, that way you can make a quick exit if necessary.

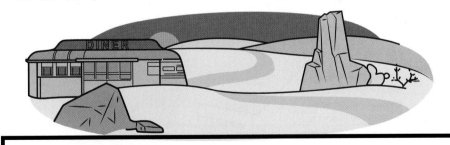

OFF-PEAK

In general, if you're going to take a baby out to eat, choose a place that's not in the thick of things, and/or don't go during the restaurant's busiest hours. If you can't, consider hiring a sitter.

Day Care

If you've never been inside a day care, it's a good idea to take tours of your options before enrolling your child in one. Here's what to look for.

Nice and neat
Is the space organized? Make sure there are designated areas for play and learning and that those areas have cubbies or shelves in which to keep the necessary materials.

Tools of the trade
Are there enough toys and learning materials to go around? Learning to share is essential, but you don't want your kid to feel left out simply because the day care is undersupplied.

GERMS
One of the major downsides of day care is the proliferation of germs. Until your kid builds a robust immune system, it might seem like they are getting a cold every week (see pg. 204).

Window shopping
First of all, there should be windows. Natural light and good ventilation are crucial to creating a comfortable environment. Just make sure the windows have safety guards.

Safety check
Like your home, a good day care should be childproofed. You should also be able to easily spot fire extinguishers, smoke detectors and first aid kits.

Good looking out

Is there an outdoor area for play? If so, it should be enclosed and only contain play sets and equipment that are the right size for your child.

Vibe check

Does the environment feel warm and welcoming? Your child will be spending a lot of time here, so you want them to be somewhere comfortable and fun (spacious, decorated with bright colors and images, etc.).

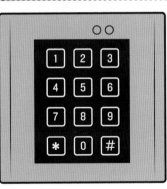

SECURITY

Any day care you tour should be routinely inspected by building safety experts. Ask the staff about their safety practices: Are doors locked at all times? Do they require photo ID and pre-approval for anyone picking up a child?

TRUST YOUR DOCTOR
While every cold doesn't mean an ER visit, a call to your pediatrician is always a good idea. Trust them to decide if an in person or virtual visit is necessary.

The Common Cold

Colds are hard to avoid, and they can be a scary event for you and your baby. Don't hesitate to call your pediatrician at the first signs of illness for some direction. The good news is that common colds are...common, and we as a species have become pretty good at finding remedies for them. It's always a good idea to have some children's Tylenol on hand, along with a dosage syringe, nasal aspirator and a NoseFrida. If you've never used the latter, don't worry; there's no risk of sucking snot into your mouth if used correctly.

1
Insert tip of nozzle into your baby's nose.

2
Suck through the mouthpiece. Mucus gets trapped in the filter.

3
Clean after use.

GET TO KNOW COMMON ILLNESSES

The world is filled with germs. Some are worse than others, and some are harder to avoid. But that's no excuse not to leave the house, and even if you could put your kid in a bubble (please don't), their immune system develops by fighting off common illnesses. Here's an intro to some that you might run into within the first year.

Conjunctivitis (pink eye) is known by the crusty, itchy and irritable eyes it produces. Prescription eye drops may be needed.

Upper respiratory infections cause runny nose, cough and fever. Monitor your child's breathing, and if they start to struggle, seek help immediately.

Influenza, COVID-19 and other forms of coronavirus are pretty much everywhere. Seek professional medical treatment and make sure your child's vaccinations are up to date.

Hand, foot and mouth disease most often affects children under 5. Symptoms include fever, rash and mouth sores. Over-the-counter pain medications can help until it clears up.

Ear infections cause ear pain, fever, irritability, difficulty sleeping and tugging at an ear. These infections are very common. Your doctor can prescribe antibiotics.

Babyproofing Basics

When you bring an infant into your home, you gain a roommate who is curious about everything yet lacks the insight to know what curiosity does to cats. In fact, babies and cats have a lot in common: They enjoy knocking things off tables, tugging on cords and climbing things they shouldn't just because they can.

When considering how best to protect your baby from your stuff, consult a checklist and do all of this before letting them loose in your home. Better yet, you can knock out many of these things during the nesting phase—that way they're already done before baby arrives.

In general

Place outlet covers over every unused outlet in your home. Even the one that doesn't seem to work anymore.

The cords on the blinds can be dangerous hazards for your kid, so cut any loops and use safety tassels and cord stops instead.

Make sure you have smoke and carbon monoxide detectors on every floor of the house, and double-check those batteries.

Medication should always live in a locked cabinet. But sometimes folks keep medicine in their purse. You don't need to demand to search any bag that comes into your home, but you should be aware when others bring in bags and ask that

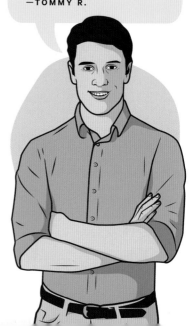

"Keep your office door closed. This space is cord city. Get that cord organizer you've been putting off buying so your space looks neat and your kid can't pull your monitor off the desk."

—TOMMY R.

LOCK YOUR DOCS

Babyproofing isn't just about keeping your kid safe from your stuff. It's also about keeping things safe from your kid, whose budding curiosity might extend to questions like "What happens if I pour milk all over these birth certificates?" Consider investing in a fireproof safe for important documents. If it can protect your passport from a fire, it'll keep your kid from flushing it down the toilet.

they place them somewhere baby couldn't possibly reach.

If you live in a home with stairs, install a baby gate.

Plastic doorknob guards are a smart idea once baby can walk.

Living room

Have a sick flat screen? Mount it. If you have a more conventional television, make sure it's situated on low, sturdy furniture.

Secure top-heavy furniture to the wall using brackets or braces (which your furniture likely came with and you may have in a junk drawer somewhere. While you're at it, clean your junk drawer).

Move furniture away from any windows so your budding escape artist doesn't clamber out and into the wild.

Block your fireplace to ensure your child can't escape through the chimney or get too close to an area that might have sharp edges. Speaking of sharp edges...

Add edge and corner guards to any furniture to prevent head injuries if your kid takes a tumble (they will).

Kitchen/laundry room

Cook on the back burners to prevent pots from being pulled down while in use. Consider installing a stove guard to avoid accidents that involve hot burners.

If you use it to clean, store it in a locked cabinet or a high shelf.

Vitamins and other supplements may be good for you but they're bad for your baby. Keep them locked up instead of on the counter. Yes, you might forget to take them, but that's better than taking your kid to the ER.

When you eat at the dinner table, ditch the tablecloth. Baby can pull it and ruin your meal by breaking all your plates.

Get a garbage can that locks. You don't want to pick up your baby from the landfill.

This one's easy: Knives and glass should be kept well out of the reach of your kid.

Place vomit emoji stickers on anything that could be considered poisonous. As soon as your kid is old enough to understand symbols, teach them what these mean.

Babyproofing Basics

(CONTINUED)

Your baby will be very curious about their surroundings, which is great! However, curiosity yields exploration of said surroundings, and that can lead to injuries if you're not prepared. Here's how to protect your baby from potential hazards at home.

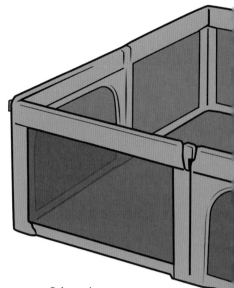

Baby enclosure

This is the ethical way to lock up your baby and spare them from getting hurt around the house. Whether you know it as a playpen, a play yard or any other name, this enclosure is great for containing your kid's crawling while you quickly take a shower or scarf down a meal.

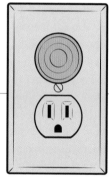

Outlet covers

The need to keep your kid safe from electricity requires no explanation. These are often considered the most essential babyproofing item.

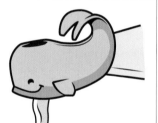

Bathtub faucet guard

Following the rule of "cover all sharp edges," it's a good idea to cover the faucet in the bathtub.

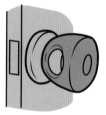

Childproof doorknob

They might not be able to reach a door knob yet, but they will...

STAIRS

If baby is crawling around the house, certain rooms or areas will be off limits due to the various potential dangers they present. Stairs, for example, should always be blocked off by a reliable baby gate.

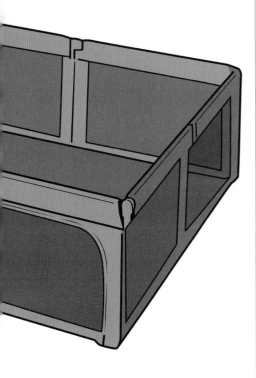

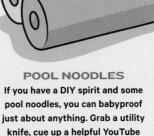

POOL NOODLES

If you have a DIY spirit and some pool noodles, you can babyproof just about anything. Grab a utility knife, cue up a helpful YouTube video and get to work.

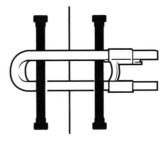

Cupboard locks

Any cupboard containing potentially harmful substances should be locked up. Added bonus: This will also stop the little one from opening all the cupboards and pulling everything out to make a huge mess.

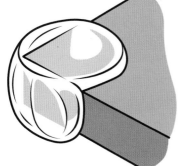

Corner guards

Babies have a knack for bumping their heads on the corners of furniture. Typically available in foam or soft rubber varieties with simple adhesives, corner guards should be placed on tables, desks and any other furniture with sharp corners.

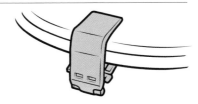

Toilet lock

If baby sees an open toilet, they might mistake it for a pool, a bath or a drinking fountain. None of those are good options. Mom will also be grateful as this will help you remember to put the seat down.

How to Speak Like a Dad

Once you become a father, it's only a matter of time before you're tasked with giving some kind of speech. When this time comes, you want to sound like you know what you're talking about (because you do!) and avoid fumbling your

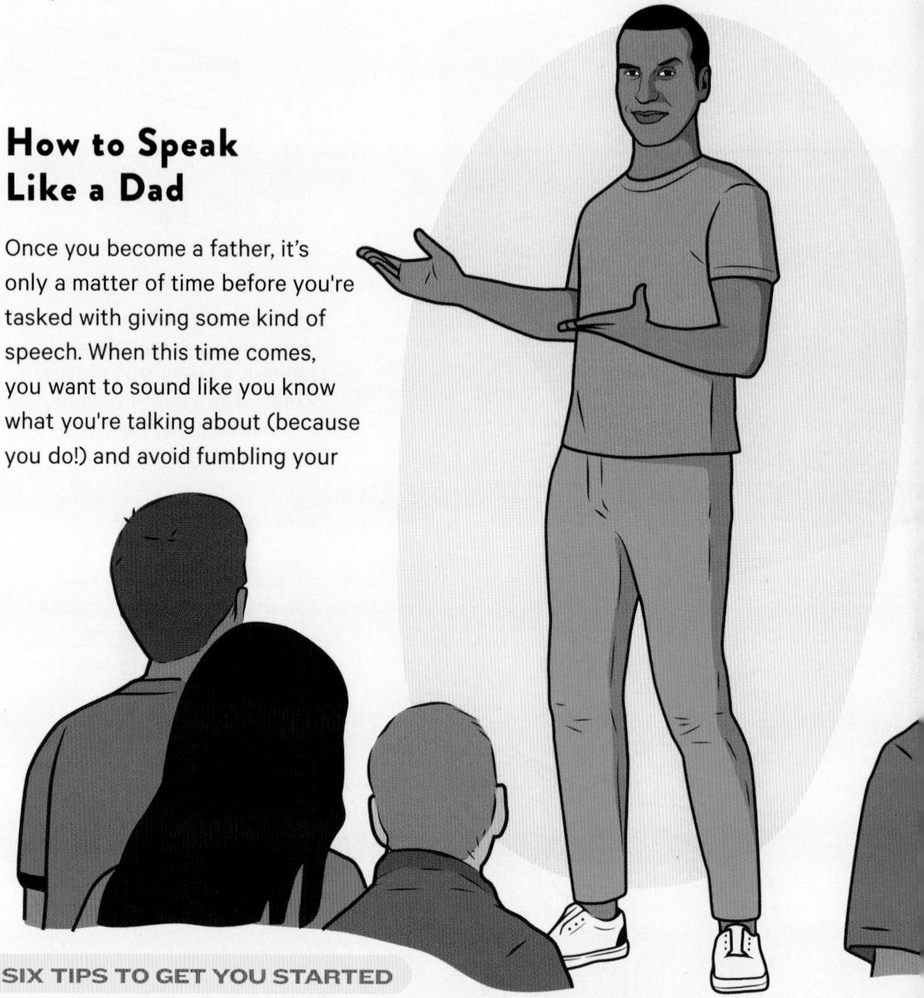

SIX TIPS TO GET YOU STARTED

(1)

Stand up

It's tough to command attention when you can't be bothered to get off your duff. Get on your feet, stand up straight and you'll feel yourself pulling focus.

(2)

Prepare your vocals

Do some voice exercises beforehand. Sing some scales, or even just gargle some mouthwash and sip some tea.

(3)

Be loud and clear

If someone yells "Can't hear you!" during your first sentence, it can kill the moment. Think of pushing your words out from your gut (read: diaphragm) as opposed to your throat to add volume.

(4)

Keep your head up

You're not trying to sink a 20-foot putt—keep your head and eyes up and read the audience for cues.

way to the point you're trying to make. Whether it's a pep talk before a big game or a toast at a wedding, here's how to captivate an audience when you need to. Or at the very least, you can make some people laugh with some well-rehearsed bathoom humor. (Do not do this.)

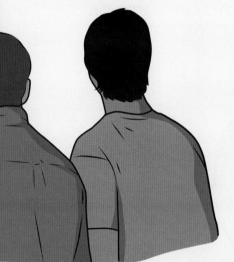

5 Joke sandwich
It's always good to start and end with a funny bit while keeping the sincere stuff as the main content in the middle. Just be aware of your setting and audience to keep it appropriate.

6 Stay on target
Identify what your goal/message is early on and keep the speech on target. Minds and ears will wander if you're rambling without making much of a point. Brevity helps.

THINGS TO AVOID:

Excessive improvising

Staring at one person

Uncontrollable crying

Reading from paper

Mumbling

Inside jokes

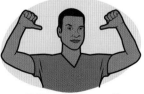

Talking about yourself

Baby Sign Language

While your kid is learning basic sounds and words, you might want to incorporate some basic sign language to work in tandem with their verbal skills. It's simple enough: Perform the hand signals whenever you say a certain word. Over time, try dropping the verbals and use only the sign. You might be surprised by how quickly your baby can pick up on things!

According to a study by Michigan State, sign language gives your baby the ability to express their needs and thoughts, which reduces their frustration and the tantrums they throw over miscommunication woes. And let's face it: Reducing tantrums is a worthwhile goal no matter what age group is involved.

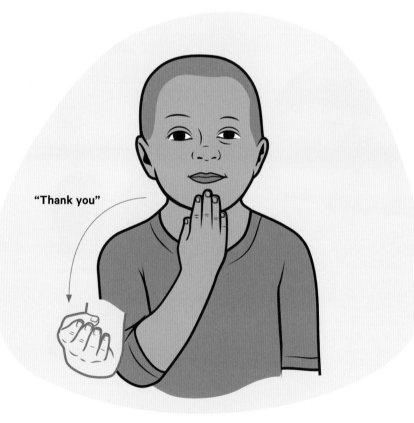

"Thank you"

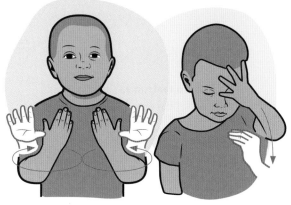

"All done" "Sleep"

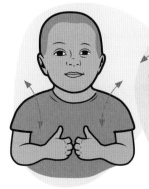

"Bath" "I love you"

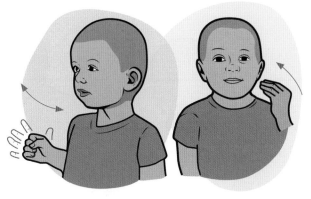

"Milk" "Eat"

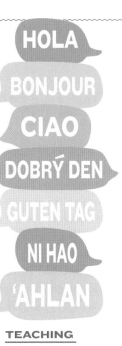

HOLA
BONJOUR
CIAO
DOBRÝ DEN
GUTEN TAG
NI HAO
'AHLAN

TEACHING A SECOND LANGUAGE

According to a Cornell University study, "Cognitive advantages follow from becoming bilingual, and these cognitive advantages can contribute to a child's future academic success." The most effective way to learn a second language, they say, is to put the young child in situations where the second language surrounds them, aka immersion.

So, if you know another language, introduce this to your child early on. If you don't, well, all the more reason to pick one and get started.

Dad-vice for the Road

Sooner or later your baby is going to start walking, running and growing faster than you can imagine. It's probably been a hell of a year, so congrats—you made it out the other side and learned a lot along the way. Maybe you're already thinking about having baby number two. Either way, time marches on, so here are 15 bits of fatherly advice to help you power through the toddler years and beyond. Enjoy the ride.

1. Let them help. Little ones learn things by doing.

2. Ignore tantrums. They don't last forever. Take a deep breath.

3. Messes can be cleaned up. These might be annoying, but as long as nobody's hurt, there's no need to lose your cool.

4. Puddles should be jumped in. Preferably with rain boots.

5. Take your kid fishing, even if you've never done it.

6. Befriend other parents with kids. You'll both have play dates.

7. Set a good example. Your child imitates you even when you least expect it.

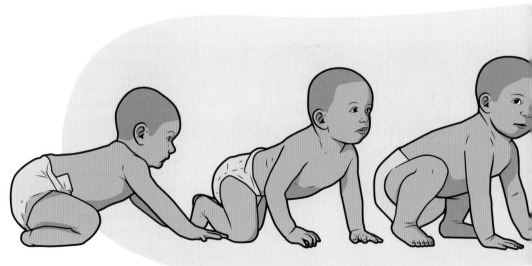

8. Listen to their words and actions. They're doing their best to communicate with you.

9. Be silly. Life's far too short to take everything so seriously.

10. Read to your child and listen to music together.

11. Perfect the zerbert and use it frequently.

12. Foster imagination and creativity, but also let your kid learn how to entertain themselves. Refrain from micromanaging their every move.

13. If something isn't working, try a different approach. There's no one-size-fits-all approach to being dad (or, for that matter, a child).

14. Encourage your child to try new things. That's how we grow.

15. Be present. Any parent will tell you it goes by in a blink. Put away the phone (unless you're taking pics or video chatting loved ones).

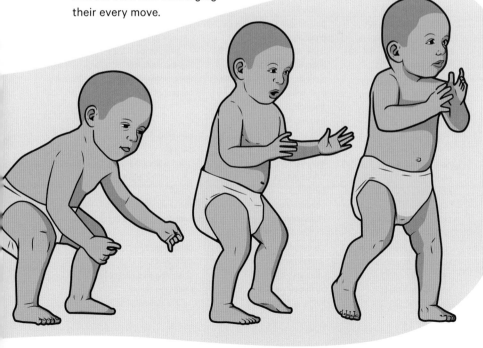

Index

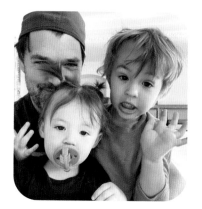

About the Author

Todd M. Detwiler is an illustrator and visual artist living just north of Detroit, Michigan. To be honest, he has few qualifications to write a book about being a dad apart from his own experience, but it turns out that's enough! He is the father of two, husband of one and happy owner of a dog named Oslo. He has worked as a caricature artist, icon designer, roofer, waiter, actor, mower-of-lawns, painter, curator, mastermind of high school prankery and wizard of peek-a-boo dark magic.

He has a website, *tmdetwiler.com*, with illustration work commissioned by *The New York Times*, *The Wall Street Journal*, Nike, Disney, Apple, Peloton and more. Todd loves to spend time working around the house and with his family, teaching his kids the difference between wants and needs, yogurt and frogurt and how to flip a pancake.

About the Experts

Vanessa Valerie Peña, MD, is a Board Certified Obstetrician and Gynecologist and a faculty member at Weill Cornell Medical College in New York City.

Amy C. Buono, MD, is a Board-Certified Pediatrician with a private practice in Millburn, New Jersey.

Acknowledgments

Writing this book wasn't easy. In fact, it was quite difficult at times. If it weren't for the help and support of some very specific people, this book would not exist. They have all my gratitude and deserve recognition.

My wife, Allie, whose patience and support is unmatched. Thank you for joining me on this journey (the book) (the kids) (life)—none of it is possible without you, and words fail to capture how much I appreciate and love you.

My kids, Teddy and Vada. You're the only inspiration I ever needed.

My mom and dad, who gave me a life filled with love and support. You raised us on a small farm in Pennsylvania with the encouragement to see a larger world beyond our own horizon.

To my brother, Chris, for braving fatherhood before me. As my older brother, I've always watched you go first and show me the way. To Brandy, Thomas and Allison, I've looked to you as a playbook for how to raise a family. You lead by example, and I will continue to look to you for guidance on how to raise quality humans.

My mother-in-law Glinda, who I'm certain would have liked this book and encouraged me to write How to Mom first, then perhaps this "Dad book thing."

To John Foster, my father-in-law. You've set a high standard as a father, one to which all dads should aspire. I know I do.

My grandfathers Thomas Detwiler Sr. and Carson Speelman Jr., and their fathers. We stand on the shoulders of those who came before us, and I have been fortunate to have a wonderful view.

My niece Ava and her two parents, Andi and James. Because of how long it took to write this book, you all served as a real-time case study (whether you realized or not).

To the experts who gave their time and knowledge to keep this book as accurate as possible, in particular Dr. Peña and Dr. Buono.

To my many friends and family who offered their experience and advice. ♥

To my publisher, Phil Sexton, who green-lit this book based on a rag-tag pitch deck held together with bubblegum and a dream.

Jeff Ashworth and Juliana Sharaf, my editors. You took a moderately literate illustrator and turned him into a writer. I deeply appreciate your patience and assistance with molding this book well beyond the author's own ability.

To every damn new dad out there. I hope this book provides you some insight, comfort and a couple laughs. There's a great responsibility in being Dad, but at its heart, it's just a lot of fun. I hope you all enjoy fatherhood as much as I do and embrace all the difficulties with patience and love. You'll make it look easy in no time.

Media Lab Books
For inquiries, call 646-449-8614

Copyright 2023 T.M. Detwiler

Published by Topix Media Lab
14 Wall Street, Suite 3C
New York, NY 10005

Printed in China

All rights reserved. No part of this book may be reproduced in any form or by any electronic or mechanical means, including information storage and retrieval systems, without permission in writing from the publisher, except by a reviewer, who may quote brief passages in a review.

The information in this book has been carefully researched, and every reasonable effort has been made to ensure its accuracy. Neither the book's publisher nor its creators assume any responsibility for any accidents, injuries, losses or other damages that might come from its use. You are solely responsible for taking any and all reasonable and necessary precautions when performing the activities detailed in its pages.

Certain photographs used in this publication are used by license or permission from the owner thereof, or are otherwise publicly available. This publication is not endorsed by any person or entity appearing herein. Any product names, logos, brands or trademarks featured or referred to in the publication are the property of their respective trademark owners. Media Lab Books is not affiliated with, nor sponsored or endorsed by, any of the persons, entities, product names, logos, brands or other trademarks featured or referred to in any of its publications.

ISBN-13: 978-1-948174-90-9
ISBN-10: 1-948174-90-1

CEO Tony Romando

Vice President & Publisher Phil Sexton
Senior Vice President of Sales & New Markets Tom Mifsud
Vice President of Retail Sales & Logistics Linda Greenblatt
Chief Financial Officer Vandana Patel
Manufacturing Director Nancy Puskuldjian
Digital Marketing & Strategy Manager Elyse Gregov

Chief Content Officer Jeff Ashworth
Director of Editorial Operations Courtney Kerrigan
Senior Acquisitions Editor Noreen Henson
Creative Director Susan Dazzo
Photo Director Dave Weiss
Executive Editor Tim Baker

Content Editor Juliana Sharaf
Features Editor Trevor Courneen
Assistant Managing Editor Tara Sherman
Designers Glen Karpowich, Mikio Sakai
Copy Editor & Fact Checker Madeline Raynor
Junior Designer Alyssa Bredin Quirós
Assistant Photo Editor Jenna Addesso

Contributing Editor Vanessa Peña, M.D.
Contributing Editor Amy Buono, M.D.

Indexing by Meridith Murray

1C-K22-1